"Suzanne Loebl's story is a poignant portrait of a mother's unconditional love rising above the tragedy of an illness that brought the end of life to her son and to so many of his generation. A must read for anyone who has cared for or lost a family member to AIDS."

—Robert B. Saper, MD, Boston University School of Medicine

"Suzanne Loebl is our guide on this journey into the hellish world of AIDS from the late 70s to the early 90s....when Suzanne joined the Mothers' Group we meet women whose stories rend the heart. Because Loebl is such a great writer, the fears, hopes, anger, desperation and self-accusation of these women reach the reader in their full force...in the end, it is the sheer humanity of the AIDS sufferers and the mothers that make this book memorable.

—George McCauley, Teacher, Theologian, Author of *Eddies Dream*

"The Mothers' Group takes us on a journey with a group of devoted mothers in their struggle to cope with the AIDS illness in their respective families. It is a story that shows the courage and love of mothers for their children, and the sensitivity, compassion and support these mothers provide to each other during the most difficult times, including the death of their children. The lives of the author and her gay son, who eventually dies of AIDS, are described in detail, as they confronts his illness yet remain determined to enjoy life to the fullest. This inspirational book reminds us of what is truly valuable in our lives.

—Phyllis Steinberg, President, PFLAG NYC

"The Mothers' Group brings together women of diverse backgrounds sharing virtually identical difficult situations to share support and tears. While emphasizing these common bonds between strangers, the story also provides an enlightening insight into the symptoms, treatment—and heartbreak—of AIDS in the 1980s and 1990s. Members of other support groups will recog-

nize the almost universal sense of guilt shared by parents and families of children facing some of life's most difficult problems, as well as the wonderful support offered by the Mothers' Group. Their acceptance of their gay children enabled them to love their children without reservation and support them through their too-short lives. Their grief was unencumbered by guilt.

—Dave Parker, Director PFLAG

"Courageous mothers have been at the front against AIDS from the beginning of the epidemic over 25 years ago, These seemingly ordinary moms advocated powerfully, forcefully and passionately for the dignity of their adult children and all children living with HIV/AIDS. The Mothers' Group is a timely chronicle of the legacy of support that these women have helped to create."

—Marjorie J. Hill, PhD, Interim Executive Director, Gay Men's Health Crisis.

"The Mothers' Group' reveals to the reader the story of those who were infected and affected by AIDS…For the mothers, families and friends anticipating grief and the bereavement the book shares that intimate journey. It is a story of courage and realism and the sharing of how 'gradually we fought our way back to emotional stability.' I hope the story will help many who are still frozen in their grief. I'm sure they will find it hard to read and it will bring up much pain, but it is in itself a vehicle of healing. I can attest to that."

—Ruth Hall, Sister of the Community of Saint Francis Director, The Family Link

The Mothers' Group

The Mothers' Group

◆

Of Love, Loss, and AIDS

Suzanne Loebl

ASJA Press
New York Lincoln Shanghai

The Mothers' Group
Of Love, Loss, and AIDS

ASJA Press
an imprint of iUniverse, Inc.

iUniverse books may be ordered through booksellers or by contacting:

iUniverse
2021 Pine Lake Road, Suite 100
Lincoln, NE 68512
www.iuniverse.com
1-800-Authors (1-800-288-4677)

The views expressed in this work are solely those of the author and do not necessarily reflect the views of the publisher, and the publisher hereby disclaims any responsibility for them.

ISBN-13: 978-0-595-41575-5
ISBN-10: 0-595-41575-X

Printed in the United States of America

Contents

PREFACE AND ACKNOWLEDGEMENT....................ix

CHAPTER 1   THE RABBIT HOLE........................1

CHAPTER 2   CALIFORNIA 17

CHAPTER 3   THE MOTHERS GROUP 26

CHAPTER 4   "GIVE ME THE STRENGTH"...............37

CHAPTER 5   AIDS IS CRAZY MAKING 47

CHAPTER 6   TO WISH UPON A STAR 81

CHAPTER 7   TWILIGHT 90

CHAPTER 8   ARMAGEDDON........................95

CHAPTER 9   MOUNT ZION.......................108

CHAPTER 10   GRIEF 122

CHAPTER 11   PROMISES TO KEEP 135

PREFACE AND ACKNOWLEDGEMENT

Nothing ever is as exhausting as denying a calamity when it stares you in the face. In 1983, a few months after he arrived in California, David, my son, had developed a brief flu-like illness. We tried to forget about the episode, though even then doctors suspected that the first symptom of an HIV/AIDS infection usually was such a "flu." Four years later the time for denial was over. There was no doubt that AIDS virus was destroying David's health.

The new, fatal illness had arrived in the United States in 1979. For many years it completely mystified the medical profession. In 1984 scientists identified the causative virus, but there were no drugs to tame it and most of those afflicted died.

I had vowed to let my children go when they were grown, but this fatal disease catapulted me right back into the center of my son's life. I was determined that I would be there for him, if he wanted my help, which he did. There are no road maps for such journeys. It required all the strength, diplomacy, compassion, courage, honesty and deception that I could muster. The undertaking proved to be immensely rewarding, terrifying, and solitary.

Fortunately I found a group of women who shared my situation. The Mothers' Group was the brain child of Fran Herman, who knew from both professional and personal experience that during crises women usually assume the brunt of caring for all the members of the family, while lacking much support of their own.

Fran's group filled a need. In 1986 a sole woman had shown up at the initial meeting. Six months later, when I joined, I was the forty-third mother to avail herself of the group's warmth and wisdom. Eventually a rotating number of about fifteen women showed up at the weekly sessions and during its eight-year long existence, the group welcomed 350 women.

The Mothers Group made me feel less lonely. It did not alter the reality of AIDS, nor the terror of knowing that my son was fatally ill. It is hard to recall the anxiety and fear of these years, or the love, joy and laughter David and I shared. It was as if the umbilical cord had grown back and reached from where I was living in New York to David's home in San Francisco.

But this is not only my story. It is the chronicle of a group of women who helped their children fight against terrible odds. It is the story of a disease that baffled and humbled the medical community. It is the tale of the American gay community as it grew to adulthood, and most of all it is a love story of a son and his mother.

Though this book centers on how I experienced the years of David's illness I want to stress that we both had our separate lives. Our existence was filled with other people who helped each of us navigate through this crisis, surrounded us with their love and keenly experienced his illness and my ultimate loss. If my book offers some insight into the mysterious ways in which one overcomes death and grief it will have achieved its purpose.

Today tens of millions need fortitude facing AIDS. When the disease entered my life it affected only a handful of people, mostly gay or intravenous drug users. Since society considers these groups marginal, no great effort was expended to stop the disease. By the time scientists, physicians, educators and epidemiologists marshaled their forces, the disease had spread around the world. It had returned to Africa where it had originated, with a vengeance, affecting 25 million people and leaving 12 million AIDS orphans. It spread to Asia, South America, Russia and China, which denied its presence for so long. By now every single country in the world has its infected population of gays, straights, men, women and children—40 million in all. So far AIDS has killed 20 million persons, including half a million in the United States.

Even though HIV/AIDS can now be controlled successfully, the drugs are so expensive that in developing countries only one patient out of six receives adequate treatment.

◆   ◆   ◆

It took me years to write The Mothers' Group. I want to thank each and every member of the group—whether mentioned by name, pseudonym or not at all—for having stood by my side during this, the most difficult part of my life. The material pertaining to the sessions of the group was written at the time they occurred. Some of this writing was amplified in personal interviews with some of the members. For reasons of continuity, the stories of individual mothers and their children have been rearranged and telescoped. In many cases additional details were obtained during one-on-one interviews. To insure the privacy of some members, names and personal details have been altered. The stories of the following are reported on in greater detail: Susan Katz and Daniel Katz; Beverly Rotter and Iris de la Cruz; Rhea Parham and Adam Balzano; Lynn and Paul; Blanche Mednick and Brian Misciagna; Beryl Aaron and Howard Aaron; Priscilla Reed and Rob Reed; Lucy and Philip; Maggie Jessup and Patrick Jessup.

I want to thank Rhea Parham Cohen, Deane Dixon, Blanche Mednic, and Beverly Rotter for being particularly helpful. Enormous thanks are also due to Fran Hermann, who founded the group, Frank Donnelly, and Susan Katz, who facilitated it for so many years. Frank, the only male member, was probably the most beloved among those who attended. Years after the group had disbanded Frank counseled many of us in his cozy digs in Chelsea. Typically, after 9/11 he provided emergency grief counseling near the site of the collapsed World Trade Towers, only to die in his sleep on September 13th, 2001.

I also want to thank my family and David's many friends for making the unbearable more bearable during his illness and after his death. Special thanks are due to Stewart Mittler, and Judy Loebl, for letting me reproduce the text of their eulogies, Naomi Gordon-Loebl for her poem, *Legacy*, The Alfred Publishing Company for use of the lyrics of "*Hello in There,*" by John Prine, Rabbi Alvin Fine for his *A Sacred Pilgrimage*, Marsha Kaleko for her poem *Almost a Prayer* and Kathryn Lance for a fine editing job.

I cannot imagine weathering this storm without the love of my husband, Ernest, with whom I shared the experience, my daughter Judy, who was extremely close to her brother, her partner John Gordon, and their children Ana, Naomi and Sean Gordon-Loebl. Each of these had their own close relationship with David; the book you hold in your hands simply celebrates mine.

LEGACY

I was five the year my uncle
died of aids. really it wasn't the aids
that killed him but the pneumonia
but we say he died of aids because
if I said that he died of pneumonia you'd say
what? No one dies of pneumonia and you wouldn't be wrong.

and sometimes I want to say yeah—it is wrong.
people shouldn't die of aids my uncle
shouldn't have been buried in front of his mother if you say
sorry, it's not enough but if you don't know what to say about
     aids
it's okay because I don't either and I was restless because
I was five and I didn't even know what pneumonia

was. but that's okay too pneumonia
has a silent p and I knew something was wrong
as the black dirt hit I couldn't see because
I was too short but my uncle
was encased in ceramic that my grandfather carried aids
to him followed and me feeling to far to say

what I really wanted to say
which was, what's going on? and what is pneumonia?
and how long are you out of school with aids?
and why does it feel so wrong
to sit in this apartment seemingly dead? and why did my uncle
leave behind his gumballs? I am wondering because

I think I'd like to eat them but they are stale because
it's cold and if someone lived here would it be heated? I wanted
     to say
these things and maybe get an answer maybe from my uncle
I thought I was old fairly sure I understood but pneumonia

is something you don't get. and I didn't get it did not want to be
    wrong

about my understanding. I thought he'd come back and say aids

wasn't so bad after all, that aids

killed him but death was just an absence because

he'd be coming back he always did every few months even if we
    had the wrong

flight number he'd still show up at the gate eventually and say

hi girls. I only knew him with a suitcase never with pneumonia

so I have to think his flight was just delayed. my uncle

should have known me, aids shouldn't have known him and we
    say

he's still with us because it's easier than saying the silent p in
    pneumonia

but wrong—the truth? all the fresh gumballs left with my uncle.

Naomi R. Gordon-Loebl

1

THE RABBIT HOLE

I had barely listened when the man gave me directions to come to the Mothers' Support Group organized by the People With AIDS Coalition. "We meet at 67 A West 11 Street. Ring bell # 2. We'll buzz you in. The door sticks…Enter the corridor…"

I had rung the bell, fumbled with the door, then entered a long, dark tunnel which reminded me of the rabbit hole of Alice in Wonderland. AIDS, with its unwritten script, was certainly scarier than any wonderland Lewis Carroll could have conjured up.

The passageway ended in a small, magic garden, the front yard of a narrow, two-story private house. I entered a living room that still radiated with the warmth of happy memories. My mouth was dry with apprehension.

A few women were exchanging small talk. New arrivals were greeted with hugs. I knew that each one of these women had a child infected by the AIDS virus. Their hearts must have been breaking, yet they looked remarkably cool and competent.

At six o'clock sharp, Fran Herman, the co-facilitator of the group, asked the ten of us to form a circle, hold hands, close our eyes and think of what had been hardest during the past week. Then we introduced ourselves and named the person we were here for. One by one the women spoke:

"I am Arlene. I am here for Barry, who has AIDS."

"I am Marion. I am here for my son, Tom."

"I am Mary. I am here for Tommy, who is HIV positive."

"I am Elaine, my daughter is ill."

"My name is Erica. I lost my son, Gary, a month ago,"

My turn came. "I am here for David, my son, who is HIV positive." How hard it had been to say that out loud. It was as if I had condemned him to death. I wanted to run, to escape; yet part of me knew that I had to stay.

Despair, pain, and loneliness had prompted me to call the Gay Men's Health Crisis (GMHC) hotline to find people with whom to share my heartache and anxiety. It had taken fortitude to dial the number, for even something as non-committal and anonymous as a phone call meant that my dread was grounded in reality.

After the formal preamble, Fran invited each woman to speak, to share small victories and defeats. Each mother talked about her child. I was too upset to concentrate, but gathered that:

Paul was responding to megavitamin therapy.

Tommy was able to return to his own apartment.

Freddy refused to speak to his mom.

Dr. Greene was a kind and caring AIDS doctor.

Barry's Hodgkins disease was in remission. Arlene, the group's medical expert, said there was a promising new drug.

Erica read a poem she had written about phoning her dead son and listening to his cheerful message on the answer machine.

Deane's ex "pulled some more shit."

The memorial for Rick was to be next Thursday.

Frank Donnelly, a gay psychotherapist to whom I had spoken on the phone, said that his friend Andy was doing poorly.

I was getting a crash course in AIDS: pain, love, hope, despair, frustration, hard work, devotion, helplessness, and most of all incredible courage. How could they stand it? I wondered.

◆   ◆   ◆

On the eve of Memorial Day, 1987, as I was preparing to join my husband Ernest in Maine, my Manhattan telephone rang. It was David.

"I did not know whether to call you," he said, "but I have bad news." He had gone to see Steven Marks, his San Francisco physician, who found that the AIDS virus had started to destroy his immune system.

I had tried to brace myself for such a phone call for a long time, but it still took me by total surprise. I wondered whether I was hearing right. Panic engulfed me. My heart pounded, my legs felt like jelly, I sank onto the rickety chair next to the phone. I willed my voice to be calm and reassuring: "Hmm," I said. "You have to do something. Perhaps you can get AZT, that new drug everybody is talking about." We chatted a bit, then "kissed" good night.

◆   ◆   ◆

Some catastrophes arrive with a bang. AIDS, a calamity that was to change my life and that of my family, had sneaked upon the world with barely a whisper. In 1981, newspapers reported that doctors had noted a sharp increase in the incidence of some unusual diseases. One was *Kaposi's sarcoma*, an exceedingly rare type of skin cancer, characterized by wine-colored, unsightly lesions. Another was *pneumocystis carinii pneumonia (PCP)*, rarely encountered in healthy people. The third was *toxoplasmosis*—a fatal infection usually found in birds and cats. Those affected died after horrible suffering. One common link between the patients was that most were gay men, and all had a severely depressed immune system. At the time there were only a few dozen cases.

Physicians started to speculate about the nature of these disorders. Were they related? Were they sexually transmitted? Did glue sniffing or some other odd behavior pattern cause them? By 1983 the guessing was over. Robert Gallo, of the National Institutes of Health in Washington, and Luc Montagnier, of the Pasteur Institute in France, discovered that a novel virus caused the disease. Once it infected a person, the virus survived by killing the cells of the immune system. The virus was named the human immune deficiency virus (HIV), and the disease it caused was called the Acquired Immune Deficiency Syndrome, or AIDS. The discovery led to the development of a reliable diagnostic test called the HIV ELISA Test.

Doctors had been relieved when the virus was identified. The effective control of infectious diseases by means of vaccines or antibiotics was, and still is, medicine's proudest achievement. The HIV virus, they felt, would be tamed rapidly.

Early in the course of this mysterious epidemic, long before the disease had a name, scientists at the Center for Disease Control (CDC) in Atlanta noted that the so-called "gay cancer" followed the transmission pattern of hepatitis. This meant that the disease was transmitted by blood and other body fluids. It could therefore be spread by sexual intercourse, blood transfusions or contaminated intravenous needles. The CDC summarized its conclusions in a report and sent it to the White House. Regan Republicans believed the news to be politically damaging, and suppressed it.

Indeed, some segments of the American population felt that gays and drug users had AIDS coming to them. Didn't the Bible explicitly condemn homosexuality? Hitler had gassed homosexuals along with the Jews and gypsies, and even the government of the United States still forbade gays and lesbians to serve openly in its Armed Forces. Believing that the majority of Americans were anti-gay, Washington did not attempt to contain the epidemic.

The Feds were not the only ones who failed to act. There also was overconfidence on the part of the medical establishment and defiance on the part of the gay community, who saw the recommended cautiousness as interference with their hard-won liberation. By the time AIDS was taken seriously, the new virus had been widely disseminated.

Even though at first the "gay cancer" seemed to be merely a medical curiosity, I worried because David was gay. I told myself not to be paranoid. Homosexuality was said to affect ten percent of the population, and I reasoned that not every gay man could be at risk.

◆   ◆   ◆

I had always hated to discuss sex with my two children; nevertheless, I talked with David about AIDS. Even the incomplete reports suggested that the plague was transmitted via sexual intercourse. Both Judy, his sister, and I pleaded with him "to be careful." David said that he knew more about AIDS than we did and recommended that we mind our own business. Besides, he reassured us, he was not very promiscuous. I shut up. In retrospect I wish that I had carried on and screamed. By the time most gay men switched to "safer sex," the disease had infiltrated the entire gay community. By 1983, when more reliable information was available, it was a matter of chance whether a particular person had been infected or not.

Almost from the beginning, David suspected that he was infected with the AIDS virus. In 1983, soon after he had arrived in San Francisco, he had a brief affair with Charles H., who worked for Pacific Bell. Within weeks, David had developed severe flu-like symptoms. At the time nobody had linked this brief illness with the mysterious disease. However, as more information became available, David realized that his "flu" probably meant that the HIV virus had infected him. I too had good reason to be suspicious. During one of my visits to California we had gone swimming. David asked me to palpate his neck. His lymph glands were markedly swollen. "You must be coming down with a cold," I told him. "No," he said, "I have lymphadenopathy (swollen lymph glands). Many gay men have it."

Since Ernest and I dutifully read any news story concerning AIDS, the information rang a bell. Doctors were concerned about the rising incidence of swollen lymph glands among homosexual men. Some scientists believed the swellings were caused by a separate mysterious disease, one that even protected those affected from developing more advanced immuno-suppression, while others saw lymphadenopathy as an early symptom of AIDS.

I had tried hard to bury the full impact of all this information, but could not forget it. Whether I was aware of it or not, AIDS was always with me. At parties I would suddenly withdraw into myself. Fear woke me in the middle of the night. How I wished that I truly believed in God. Why was this happening to me? I imagined David tethered to machines in a hospital bed. I had weird dreams. I hoped that I would be dead before I had to deal with the reality of this disaster. When the stress became too intense, taking advantage of the time difference between New York and California, I called David. His small talk about his friends, his roommates, and his classes reassured me.

David's 1987 Memorial Day phone call told me that the time for fantasy games was over. Until then I had no concrete evidence that the virus had infected David so I could—partially—deny facts. Now there was no longer any escape. I had to let AIDS into my life. I had been awakened from a deep slumber and could not get back to sleep. I tried to read, but could not concentrate. I took a sleeping pill. It did not help. I drank some gin, half hoping the combination would do me in. Still no sleep! The drugs and the liquor simply made me feel worse. Day finally dawned and I staggered to the airport and onto my plane. I was a mess.

Twenty years earlier my husband and I had bought an old summer cottage on Echo Lake on Mount Desert Island. It was our escape from city life. When the children were small we spent our summers hiking, swimming, and reading. Even after they were grown, Judy and David visited each year, walking the Maine woods with their friends and lovers.

Spring in Maine is magic. The woods that hug the cottage are filled with pink ladies slippers. Lilac perfumes the whole island and vast expanses of lupines color the meadows. The ocean glistens, the waves crash against the rocks. "Yes," the world seemed to say: "I am majestic. Celebrate my radiance, bask in my peace, delight in being here."

That spring, Maine's beauty mocked my distress. I was restless, cried, got annoyed at my husband, and was glad to escape nature's glory and return to drabber Manhattan, where my everyday routine left me less time to be terrified.

◆   ◆   ◆

I was half awake when David was born on February 19, 1956. I squirmed as Dr. Kuntze, my obstetrician, stitched me up. "Look at your son," an attending resident said to distract me. There he was, my son, so little, so frail, so pale, and so helpless. A brand new human being! He beat the air with his little arms and legs. I bonded to him, and ever since he has lived in my heart, sparking stronger feelings of joy, grief and rage than anyone else in my life.

Through the haze of the anesthesia I heard Dr. Kuntze asking the nurse to leave the baby in the delivery room so he could examine him. "I'll let the pediatrician take care of it," he finally declared.

Why did anyone have to worry about my baby? I wondered. I was frightened, but too sleepy and weak to inquire. Anxiously, I waited until the next morning, when Kuntze came to see me. The doctor was sorry that I had overheard his remark. He said that after the delivery he noticed that David's tongue seemed a bit flat. Indeed, closer inspection revealed a partial tongue tie, which Kuntze felt would not interfere with the baby's sucking. Further attention proved unnecessary.

I must have been preconditioned to worry about my son, because the incident stuck in my mind. My mom had said that every mother has one *Sorgenkind,* a child about whom she worried more than about the others. I assumed that David was going to be mine.

Childbirth during the 1950's was light years away from what it is today. There was no Lamaze training. Women were anesthetized during delivery; fathers were relegated to the waiting room and babies were fed from a bottle. Those who insisted on breast-feeding their babies had to wing it on their own.

It had taken a long time before Judy nursed comfortably. It was much easier to breast-feed my second child. David and I hit it off from the start. It was clear that David loved to eat. It was a very special time for both of us. When David and I came home from the hospital, Judy welcomed her little brother with open arms.

Birth is such a miracle that parents find reasons to believe that their children are special. My husband Ernest and I certainly did. Both of us were born in Europe, he in Austria, I in Germany. During our youth our own lives had been overshadowed by the Holocaust.

I was eight when the Nazis came to power in Germany. When I was 12, my family escaped to Belgium. Two years later the Nazis invaded our refuge. My father was deported to Southern France. From there he managed to escape to the United States. My mother, now a single parent, my sister and I spent a long four years avoiding being sent to an extermination camp. I survived as a mother's helper, working for a succession of Belgian families who risked their lives to save mine. In spite of the horror of the Holocaust, their generosity endowed me with a deep faith in humanity.

Still, the chaos that had surrounded my youth had made me wary. Years earlier I had doubted that my life would be normal enough to include respectable citizenship, a husband, a household of my own, and friends.

Now I was overjoyed to have a daughter and a son. My family valued boys more than girls. My grandmother still regretted that she had not produced a male heir, and my mother had been openly disappointed that she too only had daughters. Giving birth to a boy seemed like an achievement on my part. I felt a bit sheepish about being glad to best my mother and grandmother. After all, there was nothing wrong with me—a mere female—or my own highly competent daughter. Yet once David was born, it felt good to talk about "my son."

We lived in a large apartment house in uptown Manhattan, which was full of young families like ours. We forged lifelong friendships. Because none of us had much money, we organized a small nursery that provided the children with playmates and the mothers with some free time. I used mine to do scientific translations and abstracts. The money I made paid for small luxuries. More important, I hoped to build these skills into a respectable, challenging occupation.

My mom had been the deciding factor in my trying to have a career. Nature had showered my mother with gifts. She wrote poetry, painted, sewed, and was a masterful storyteller. She was truly beautiful and could charm birds out of trees. When she was young, few women had a profession, and she never developed any of her talents. She was not unhappy. In Hanover she hobnobbed with the city's small artistic community, and she was content. World War II disrupted her life. Shortly after we arrived in New York in 1946 my father died, leaving her a widow at 48. My mom was not equipped to have a glamorous job, and she was too well off to take a menial one. She was frustrated, lonely and bored, and relied heavily on me for her amusement.

I was determined not to repeat my mom's pattern. The war had frequently interrupted my studies. I never completed my graduate education in chemistry. Instead of going back to school, I used my training and became a science writer. It was a serendipitous decision. In 1957 the Russians had launched Sputnik, and the United States discovered a need for people who could explain scientific developments to lay audiences. My career provided me with many of the perks my mother never had: recognition, money of my own, a purpose, colleagues, and travel. My mother's reaction was ambivalent. Though she was proud of my achievement, she was also envious. I understood her conflicted feelings. I hid from her, and even from myself, the hard work it had taken to achieve what I had, and I de-emphasized my actually quite modest success.

Undistorted by emotional conflicts, my mother's relationship with my children was simple. She was an exciting grandmother. They humored her peculiarities and recognized her strengths. For David she was a welcome ally against parental oppression.

Ernest was born in Vienna. He had been a miracle baby, the only child of a 42-year old mother and a 50-year old father. He was everything his aging parents could have wished for. He was unusually bright, precocious, conscientious, and trustworthy. Nevertheless, something must have been amiss. He fantasized about being invisible, orphaned, and abandoned. He feared loss and rejection, forestalling the hurt by avoiding emotional intimacy. In 1938 the Loebls escaped to Israel.

There Ernest went to the Hebrew University, majoring in chemistry. He arrived at New York's Columbia University in 1947 to obtain his doctorate. One day we met in the library. He was brilliant, attractive, knowledgeable, and much fun to be with. I also sensed a vulnerability that appealed to my mothering instincts. We spent a weekend together in Tanglewood during the summer of 1949, and knew that this was it. We shared a love for the outdoors, the theater, music, going to museums, travel and eating good food.

We were married in 1950. After Ernest's graduation he was appointed as a professor at the Polytechnic University of New York. He never returned to Israel, and in time would view his remaining in the United States as a betrayal of the feisty, newborn state that had sheltered him from the Holocaust.

Even when my passion for Ernest was at its most intense, I was aware of his emotional baggage. For many years I believed that my love would overcome his problems. And indeed many aspects of our marriage were good. Our youth had been so traumatic that both of us needed the security and strength our union provided.

I often acted as a buffer between Ernest and the outside world. The arrangement seemed to suit the two of us, except that it enabled Ernest to remain walled off in his ivory tower, and sometimes left me feeling lonely and isolated. I was the proverbial power behind the throne, a state of affairs that echoed the philosophy of one of my great-grandmothers, who was reported to have said: "I kept all the unpleasant news to myself, but when Isaac had to know, I told him when he was in the bath, so that he could not run away."

Having Judy and David completed our family. Our son was not an easy child to raise. He had definite ideas about right and wrong, and his concepts were often at variance with mine. He had unrealistic expectations of his friends, and since life is often unfair, felt frequently dissatisfied. He was extremely loyal, and stood up when he believed that someone was wronged. He felt that I too was in need of protection, and he confronted his sometimes rash and impatient father. David was jealous of his sister, but loved her very much. He always insisted on what he thought was his due.

None of that, however, affected the special bond I shared with my son. Nobody has ever figured out how and why relationships develop. Was I responding to David's love and need? Was he sensing my deep devotion, my joy and gratitude at being a mother? Were we sharing the same lust for life, and a common sense of humor? Whatever it was he sensed that part of me regretted having to be responsible and grown up. I still have a stuffed Steiff zebra he gave me on my birthday when he was five years old.

David did not share my delight in his being a boy. When he was about three he started to dress up consistently as a little girl. He hid his hair under a kerchief. He insisted that his name was Mary. Whenever he drew a person, she had long hair. He claimed that he could not draw boys. After this behavior persisted for a year, a friend suggested that we take him to be evaluated by a psychiatrist. During the 1960s and 70s, we all believed that psychotherapy could fix any problems, so we took David to the Jewish Board of Guardians.

After many tests and much soul-searching, it was concluded that David had a "sex-identification problem." They assigned the case to a Dr. Z., a child psychiatrist, who was to see David four times a week, Ernest and me once a week each. Dr. Z. was a kind man. He was also a pure Freudian, at a time when this school of psychiatry considered homosexuality a deviant behavior. Ernest, David and I saw Doctor Z. and other psychotherapists for several years. I do not know how much of an impact the doctor had on my two men, but he had a powerful effect on me.

After all these years, it is hard for me to understand my distress at the possibility that David might grow up to be gay. As a Jew in Germany, as a German in Belgium, as an immigrant in America, I had always been different from those around me. I had hated it. Now I longed to blend in. I wanted my children to be like everybody else's, except better. I did not want to make excuses for David.

I convinced myself that I was totally responsible for David's problems. I wondered whether I loved him too much; too little? Was I envious that he was the boy my mother had wanted instead of me? Was I incapable of properly raising the children nature had given me? Did I overprotect Judy, and was David jealous? Was I showing the world that being male was not that special? Was my professed broad-mindedness a farce, and was I a "closet homophobe?"

I usually am remarkably fit. But this crisis sapped my strength. My stomach hurt. I was tired. I slept poorly. I had headaches. I became pregnant again. I felt that I could not give birth to another child since I was incapable of bringing up those I had already. I pondered whether I had conceived because I wanted to replace David. Terminating the pregnancy would not resolve the problem, because the obscure forces I believed were ruling my life might punish me for having an abortion. In the end, with Ernest's consent, I opted for an illegal abortion, crying all the time while the doctor scraped out my uterus. I wondered whether I would ever extricate myself from this emotional quagmire.

Sometimes reason tried to prevail, and I asked myself why I didn't simply enjoy David, that delightful child fate had sent my way. He was funny, bright, aggressive, creative, and provocative. He loved music and dancing. He loved the theater, books and records. He loved people or hated them. He could drive you up the wall.

Ernest calmly accepted the possibility of David's homosexuality. "Perhaps he'll be happier that way," my husband suggested at a time when I still rejected the thought with all my might.

David's therapeutic stint at the Jewish Board of Guardians came to an end when he was seven. My husband had a sabbatical leave from his teaching job in New York and we spent a year in England. David's psychiatrist protested our interrupting the therapy, but we went anyway. It was a relief, and the year turned out to be great. Ernest and I enjoyed being back in Europe with our children. We made new friends, rubbed brasses, went sightseeing and attended little country fairs. When we returned to New York, the importance of the two years we had spent in therapy at the Jewish Board of Guardians had receded.

Our formerly solidly middle class neighborhood in Washington Heights was going downhill. Many of our friends had moved to the suburbs. We stayed, taking advantage of Manhattan's special schools and its cultural resources. David attended the local public school. He played a central role in his class, though he did not have any particularly close pals. He maintained his old nursery-school friendships, spent time with his grandmother, his sister and her friends. He became an avid theater buff, took pottery, studied the flute and was generally busy and content.

By comparison with the teenagers featured in newspaper headlines—drugs, pregnancy, excessive drinking, and dropping out of school my childrens' teens were tame. Still, my son was often obnoxious. There were endless arguments about homework, helping with the dishes, cleaning up his room, watching television, bedtime, not washing for a whole week, or monopolizing the bathroom extensively when we all needed it. His relationship with his father was particularly rocky.

Though I tried, I never understood the lack of rapport of the two most important men in my life. Actually, they shared many good and bad character traits. It was the undesirable ones that caused the trouble. Both were provocative, aggressive, and possessive. Both wanted my entire loyalty and devotion, both wanted to be in control. Both were afraid to be short-changed, and thus wanted more than their share. Both were sensitive and vulnerable. David interpreted Ernest's fear of emotional involvement as indifference and rejection, and responded by being offensive. When David was a child, the confrontations frequently had taken place at the dinner table. I remember David drowning his food in ketchup and Ernest insisting on reading the mail while the rest of us sat in silence. Later the clashes became more subtle. I trust that if it had not been for AIDS, the two eventually would have straightened out their relationship. Still, when David was a teen he was unpleasant with his father and even with me.

When David left for Brandeis University in Boston, I was relieved that he was moving out. However, we remained in close touch. David always wanted us to be involved in his life. Now he invited his college friends to visit in New York. David majored in psychology, a common 1970s copout for the undecided. His film-making minor was more promising. David moved back home during his junior year in college to study at New York University. He had become kind and helpful, he was a pleasure to be with.

When fall came and he returned to Boston, my empty nest aggrieved me, but I knew that was how it should be. Letting one's children go is an important aspect of successful motherhood. David and I strenuously avoided talking about his being gay. I hoped that the problem had resolved itself. During his college freshman year he even had a girlfriend whom he introduced to us. And yet I sensed that he certainly was hiding things from us, if not from himself.

◆   ◆   ◆

Over the years I had honed my skills as a science writer, and earned some much-needed money. I had been working from home because I wanted to be a fulltime mom. By 1967 I had written and published my first book, *The Story of Viruses*. I had been awarded a fellowship at the School of Journalism at Columbia University, and gradually felt better about my professional achievements. In 1971, I became the science editor of the Arthritis Foundation.

In 1977, the summer David graduated from Brandeis, my job took me for two weeks to San Francisco. As a graduation present I invited him to join me in California after my professional obligations were finished. We rented a car and drove up along the spectacular Northern Pacific coast to Oregon. We stopped in Point Reyes, Mendocino, and Eureka. We hiked, ate, visited wineries, took loads of pictures and forged an adult relationship. We discovered that we liked spending unhurried time together. We laughed at the same things, shared an uncanny ability to recall events that had happened eons ago, enjoyed eating in restaurants, and delighted in dissecting the psychological make-up of people we encountered.

We seldom disagreed. There had been some minor discord about David's driving too fast, or getting started in the morning. "Early," I said. "Late," David said. I remember only one major quarrel, and though we only talked about it ten years later, it centered around David's "in the closet" homosexuality.

That particular evening we ate in our hotel in Gold Beach, Oregon. The dining room adjoined the local disco. I went to bed after dinner, David stayed in the bar. I went to sleep, then woke with a start.

"Where was my son? I wondered. "Had someone offered him drugs? Sex? Seduced him? Abducted him? What was I to do if he vanished in the wilds of Oregon?"

I became increasingly distraught. I tried to tell myself that during the past four years David had lived in Boston and I had not known where he was. But nighttime is spooky, and when David returned to our room, at three AM, I screamed and carried on demanding to know what had happened He did not tell me where he had been, but said: "I should not have stayed out so late, I know how scared you get."

Years later, when David and I talked about this magical trip, including the Gold Beach incident, he told me that "the man who stared at us all through dinner," had picked him up as soon as I had gone to my room. When I told him that

I had gotten so upset because I suspected something like that, David was surprised that I had had so much insight.

Upon our return from California, David went to Provincetown, which became one of his favorite haunts. He worked as a houseboy, busboy and finally waiter. The child who had had so much trouble finding friends now was very popular. Making friends and keeping them became one of his life's great pleasures. When Provincetown shifted into its winter mode, David stayed in Boston, sharing an apartment with one man and two women he had met on the Cape. He still did not know what to do with himself. During the Christmas season, he sold books at Jordan Marsh, and was so good at it that the department store hired him for their shoe department. Relying on his psychological sensitivity and charm, he became am excellent salesman. I would have preferred him to be more goal-oriented, but figured that he could always go back to school when he was ready.

By then Ernest and I had surmised that David was gay. We had not broached the subject with him, feeling that it was up to our son to bring it up. He finally did so in 1979:

Tuesday Evening

Dearest Mommy and Daddy

This is one of the hardest things that I have ever done, yet I am relieved that I am finally doing it. You see I set it up so I had no choice in the matter and I had to tell you that I'm gay. Well there it is—its out—and although my heart is pounding like a jackhammer, nothing will erase what's down in black and white (actually blue and white). I have thought about telling you two and how it would go—no not just thought, but dreamt, had imaginary conversations, wrote letters, discussed it with innumerable friends, even tried to do it—since I decided about myself, when I was 19. Actually, I guess I was always gay; as soon as I had any sexual thoughts and fantasies, they were centered around men. That's the way it is with most gay people—"Coming out" is just accepting the truth about yourself and being happy about it.

I was so scared about telling you because I didn't want to lose your love and approval. I didn't want you to think of me as someone different from the son you loved before you knew he was a homosexual.

I rationalized not telling you by telling myself that it had nothing to do with our relationship, that our family didn't talk about such things (Judy never discusses her boyfriends etc.)—there were always a million reasons for not telling—but I want you to know now because it is a very important part of my life and honesty will hopefully serve to bring us all closer together.

I want to share with you the happiness I have found with Alan, who is my lover. We met in Provincetown on July 4th, 1977 and really fell in love at first sight. We have been together ever since (except for that month before I moved up to Allston) and we have our ups and downs, as any couple does, but he is very good for me and I for him. I would very much like for you to get to know each other. You would see that he is a very special person.

Where this goes from here is really up to you. You can be mad, hurt, curious, sad, anxious. You could ignore it. You could ignore me. You could try to understand. Just remember that I love you very much and I hope you feel the same. See you this weekend.

David

The letter had been prompted by our upcoming trip to Boston that weekend. David had invited us for lunch to the apartment he shared with his "roommate," Alan. Since there was only a double bed in the entire apartment, our son figured that he had better wise us up, hence the "coming out letter."

David being David, the letter had been mailed so late that it arrived only after our return to New York. It was just as well that we really had known all along. During that weekend I had still resisted acknowledging the fact. During the lunch, I had avoiding going into the bedroom. Ernest, however, was much more open and accepting and at about that time he and David had one of their rare open talks.

I felt curiously defeated by David's letter. Somehow I had hoped all these years that my son would fight his natural inclination, and would opt to be straight. My years with Dr. Z., buttressed by the prevailing social opinion, had insured that I would feel guilty about having raised a gay son.

Finally, however, I had done a smart thing for myself. Realizing that I needed help with my feelings, I went to see Dan Rosenblatt, a highly qualified gay psychotherapist. I would not have known that Dan was a homosexual had I not been told beforehand. I respected Dan enough to accept his opinion and to discuss my mixed reactions to David's homosexuality.

Eventually, after my son's friends became my friends and I became an honorary member of the gay community, I would be able to enjoy the special qualities of gays. At the time, however, all I needed to know was that homosexuals were just like everybody else: nice, mean, talented, stupid, generous, stingy, courageous, scared, and even prejudiced.

I never found out how Dan Rosenblatt felt about my conflicted feelings, but he volunteered that in his twenties he had "come out" to everybody except his own beloved mother. I concluded that emotionally two plus two do not always equal four. It might not be logical, but one could be at once tolerant of different lifestyles and be regretful about those adopted by one's own children. Hearing that such irrationality was rather common between mothers and their gay sons erased part of my feelings of guilt.

After he had "come out," a cloud lifted from my relationship with David. We had always been very fond of one another, but communication had been hampered by the knowledge that some things remained unsaid. Now I allowed myself to enjoy David fully. He took a child-like pleasure in little things—seeing a famous person in a restaurant, getting free tickets to a movie, solving a crossword puzzle. He knew all about movies, theaters, musicals. He could imitate every accent—including mine—and mimic his favorite actors and actresses. He devoured life in great gulps, thinking nothing of working all day and dancing half the night.

My son was proud of me: the books I wrote, the clothes I wore, the languages I spoke. I did my best to fulfill his expectations. I always willingly did more for him than for the rest of my family.

I still have a few letters from David's post-college Boston years. Rereading them now makes me realize that my "little boy" had grown into a responsible, loving man. He cared deeply about those crossing his path: his family, his old and new friends, his bosses, neighbors and coworkers. Here is his letter for my birthday:

Thursday afternoon [May 1982]

Dear M.

I am sitting in the park enjoying the tuna fish sandwich I brought with me from home. It just rained hard here, easing some of the mugginess, and now the sun is out and the birds are singing.

Spring is my favorite time of the year one just appreciates the good weather so much after having been through all that cold time. That is one reason for not moving to California. I am sure I would start taking the warmth and the sun for granted (although maybe there's nothing wrong with that.) Another reason for not moving there is the distance from the family. I see you too rarely as is, and we're only 200 miles away from one another. How often would we get together if we were 3,000 miles apart?

On the other hand, it might not be such a bad idea to go to school out there for two years to get the whole California thing out of my system.

Another idea, among many that I am toying with, is moving farther out of the city [Boston]—to a cheaper place—and buying a car. I'm scared of owning a car, but that's something I have to get over.

Alan is moving out June 1st, if all goes well, and he finds another place! I hope this separation works out for the best, whatever happens—either we decide we would be happier together or we decide we like it better apart. In any case, I'm looking forward to living by myself for the <u>first</u> time ever. It will mean not saving any money for a while, but for now there is enough in the bank. It is more important for me to decide which direction I want to move in. How well I do on the GMAT (Graduate Management Aptitude Test) will determine what schools I apply to. I want to go to a good school, but not necessarily the best—I want to excel in school this time around.

I am going to begin working on my resume. After my vacation in August I shall seriously begin to look for a new job—in the meantime I may pursue the help wanted ads in the [Boston] Globe every week. I wish the New York Times we get up here included the help wanted ads on Sunday, but it doesn't.

Another major project for the summer is getting my wisdom teeth out. Have I told you that I finally found a dentist that I like and trust as much as Gene [our friend and family dentist]. He's really good. I have my eye doctor, now all I need is a G.P. and I'll be all set (except for a shrink!)...

I guess this didn't turn out to be much of a birthday letter. I want to wish you all the happiness in the world—you deserve it—for the coming year. I decided against getting you the necklace, but will get you something extremely nice instead.

When will I see you? Memorial Day or the week after? Would you like to sleep over? Talk to you soon, I hope. Love and kisses

DAVID

David and Alan never patched up their relationship, and my son now lived alone. He soon found another love—Joseph. He was tired of selling shoes. His GMAT score were excellent and the sole business school he applied to was that of the University of California at Berkeley. Since I happened to visit on deadline day, I ended up typing the final version of the obligatory essay. Racing to the post office, we arrived just five minutes before it closed. My son's confidence had been well-founded. The University of California accepted him. David packed up his belongings and moved to Oakland. His doe-like, 50-pound dog Liza, a gift from Alan, was to follow later.

2

CALIFORNIA

David had arrived in California on August 12, 1983, a good omen since it was my father's birthday. My son was 27 years old, good looking and gay. For him San Francisco was the place to be. Or so it seemed, because actually AIDS' shadow was already dimming the California sunshine.

When David arrived in San Francisco he studied the "For Rent" ads in the local gay press. Among many choices he settled on a house share in Oakland, a short bus ride from Berkeley. His landlord, Gary—a gay high school teacher—welcomed not only David but Liza, feeling that she would be good company for Raffles, his aging Lab retriever.

Six months later, when I went to check on my student son, he and Gary met me at the airport. I was to stay at Gary's house and was a bit apprehensive about my immersion into the gay world. Indeed, when the weekend rolled around the curlers and make-up littering the bathroom upset me. Did that proper-looking high school teacher turn into a weekend drag queen? Would there be wild parties? I was of course wrong. My fears were a remnant of "straight" prejudice. To my relief and shame, I found out that the cosmetics belonged to the girls who visited another one of the roommates.

David had a knack for making friends. Gary loved him, as did other inhabitants of the house, as did his classmates in business school in Berkeley. On that first visit I met Andrea Lepcio, Dave Nelson, Lindsey Schubel, Robert Driscoll and a couple of other people, all of whom became permanent fixtures in David's life. My son and I walked around San Francisco's Castro, watching rainbow-colored flags fluttering in the wind. As the mother of a gay man, I too breathed more freely here.

I reaped the rewards of having accepted David's homosexuality. It seemed that standing by my gay child entitled me to respect. I appreciated the special sensitivity of many gays and began to understand in-jokes. As a Jew and World-War II refugee, I identified readily with the gay world's ever-present self-doubt, pride and need to prove itself.

Yet all was not well. AIDS was slowly creeping into the consciousness of the gay community. Newspaper reports about the disease increased, and even the public health departments started to view it as a threat. For most of us, however, it was still like distant thunder. Would the storm come closer? Would it change direction and go out to sea? Sometimes I stared at the gathering clouds and was transfixed by an ill-defined fear. Most often I looked in the opposite direction and dealt with everyday concerns: the textbook I was writing, caring for my demanding aged mother, running the house, training Sasha, the dachshund puppy David had given me for my sixtieth birthday. Yet at the bottom of my heart there was always dread about this terrifying new disease.

What was the nature of AIDS? When would there be a cure? Was it like syphilis? Like cancer? Like hepatitis? How was it transmitted? How fatal was it? Early on, doctors speculated that 40 percent of those affected might die. Slowly that percentage increased: 50, 60, 80, 100! My background as a science writer helped. I combed the scientific journals. There were no answers; only questions. Research was grinding away much too slowly. Still, since from 1981 on scientists assumed that the disease was sexually transmitted, it is hard to understand why this information was not screamed from the rooftops.

◆   ◆   ◆

San Francisco and business school agreed with my son. He had finally developed professional goals. He was getting top grades in his courses and was active in student affairs. He co-founded an investment club and organized a management group at whose meetings Fortune 500 companies discussed their business philosophy and employment needs. My son felt rich. He wrote:

"Give me seven years and then we can all retire in high style: Winters in Aruba or maybe Mykonos, spring in Paris, summer in Maine and fall in California sounds good to me...

David loved California's beauty, the freedom of being openly gay, of dancing non-stop at the I-Beam or other gay discos. Here is another missive from that first California year:

The weather has been so nice that its almost boring. You really would love it...The Bay is so beautiful and I cross it every time I go into San Francisco. I'm starting to want a car—I never felt I needed one before, but I do now. There is so much to see and do within a day's drive of San Fran: the wine country, Lake Tahoe, Big Sur, Carmel/Monterey, Yosemite.

There was other good news: A summer job with Pacific Bell, financial aid for the coming year, trips back East and most of all a new love. Jeff was a native Californian, the son of a professor teaching at one of the University of California's many campuses.

Handsome and upbeat, Jeff was most likable. David felt sure that he wanted to spend the rest of his life with him. Jeff was not that certain. He was in his early twenties, had just come out, and was not ready to settle down into a monogamous relationship. Emotionally he and David were at different stages of life. To prove his independence, Jeff stayed on in Sacramento, working for the California legislature.

June 1985, rolled around. David graduated from business school. Ernest, Judy—who was by then studying physical therapy at Downstate Medical Center—and I flew out to California for commencement. We went to parties, consumed fancy dinners and almost got arrested for drunken driving. We met more of David's schoolmates. Jeff participated in all our activities. The family reunion was great. David, who appreciated that his father had come all the way to celebrate his success, was gracious.

It is hard for me to describe the inner contentment I experienced when I was together with my two children. As I had resolved so long ago, I had let them go willingly and was proud that they lived their own lives without feeling excessively guilty at having left the nest. I too had my own compelling interests. And yet, when both Judy and David were with me, my entire being shifted to a new level of wholeness. It was as if I had regained a missing limb. At David's graduation I basked in contentment as I looked at Judy's finely chiseled features, David's beaming blue eyes, and listened to their cheerful chatter.

After graduation, Ernest and I made a pilgrimage to Big Sur where, for me, heaven and earth melt into one. I was humbled by nature's might. I gazed at the bare yellow hills, the precipitous cliffs, the power of the surf, the soaring birds, and came away strengthened.

The American Telephone and Telegraph Company (AT & T) had offered David a good job. He was as successful at selling telephone systems as he had been selling shoes, was good at figures, computers and sales projections. David's team won all kinds of trophies and bonuses. But David's heart never truly belonged to the phone company. His real life was dancing, movies, the theater, and friendships. He was the life of any party he attended.

In the winter of 1985 Jeff finally moved to San Francisco, but to David's disappointment he insisted on getting his own apartment. I sensed that major cracks were developing in their relationship.

By now David worried intensely about the plague. He was concerned about Jeff and his lack of health insurance. David urged Jeff to have himself tested for AIDS. Initially Jeff refused. Then, mostly to reassure his worried parents and David, he relented.

"I had very few relationships," Jeff told me much later, "I felt there was no need for concern." He was wrong. To his great surprise, Jeff turned out to be HIV-positive! The realization that his body was now a ticking time bomb shattered Jeff. He was so very young and had barely traveled outside his native state. He had to leave California and experience the world. David wanted him to stay.

The two tried to work it out for a while. At my son's insistence they even consulted a couples therapist. In the end, Jeff decided to move to Washington, D.C. My brave son gave him a big farewell party. When Jeff finally drove off, David broke down. I wondered whether he would find anybody else he loved as much ever again.

I also worried about Judy. Would she find her soul mate? Would she have children? Perhaps my apprehension had been premature. During the previous two years Judy had been seeing John Gordon, whom she had met at some leftist good cause or other. I knew Judy loved John, but their relationship was on-again, off-again. When it was off, Judy was again on her own and sad. Then there was another turn-around, and John was back in Judy's life.

I guessed most of that. We had never met John. Unlike David, who liked me to be part of every aspect of his life, Judy was rather secretive. To my immense relief, Judy and John finally decided to make a permanent go of it. Though they never legalized their relationship, it seemed solid enough for them "to live happily forever after."

We met John and liked him. With his wild, curly hair, he looked like a member of our family, except that Judy's ancestors were short and John was over six feet tall. John was Irish and Catholic and one of seven children, including two sets of twins. Winter, 1986, Judy told us that she was expecting twins!

David was proud of his sister and much relieved that she was pregnant. He felt that I deserved grandchildren and doubted that he would be a parent. As he put it, Judy's news took a great load off his mind.

◆   ◆   ◆

AT & T had provided David with a choice of health care options. David had selected a Kaiser-Permanente HMO. It had taken him months to find Steven Marks, a gay primary care physician. Now David was disenchanted with him. By the mid 1980's, AIDS was the number one concern of the gay community, yet Marks had never bothered to confirm or rule out David's HIV status. Perhaps Marks genuinely believed that AIDS was so hopeless there was no point in knowing. Perhaps he felt that a positive test result would upset David. My son, however, was action minded, and he wanted Marks to evaluate his immune function, especially his T-4 lymphocytes.

At that time, the number of T-4 cells (one subgroup of white blood cells) were a measure of the progression of the infection from non-symptomatic to full-blown AIDS. Even today such a count is the gold standard by which disease activity is measured. Marks dragged his feet about ordering a T-4 count, arguing that the test was expensive and useless, since there were no drugs to halt the inevitable downward spiral of the disease.

By 1987, this was fortunately no longer quite true. The previous year scientists had dusted off zidovudine (AZT), an old-anti-cancer drug that seemed to slow the destruction of the immune system. The drug unfortunately was extremely toxic, expensive and hard to come by. News concerning this first anti-AIDS drug was hushed up. For years nobody knew whether AZT was effective, but it was the only game in town.

Eventually my son convinced Dr. Marks to perform a T-4 cell count, whose unfortunate results David had reported that 1987 Memorial Day eve. At the time he had 450 T-cells, instead of the normal 800–1500! The count was the first indication that the AIDS virus had begun to destroy David's immune system.

In spite of his reluctance, Dr. Marks was now trying to obtain some AZT for David. We crossed our fingers. Within weeks Marks succeeded and David was on AZT. The drug had to be taken every four hours, preferably round the clock. David bought a pill-minder that rang whenever it was time to take another dose. Its chime was a constant reminder of the deadly virus. My heart skipped a beat whenever I heard it. For those in the know, the alarm was a dead giveaway: to others it was a puzzle. David was horrified whenever the pill-minder rang while he was talking to someone at work.

◆   ◆   ◆

Julian Worth, my cousin's son, was getting married in Scotland in June, two months before Judy's babies were due. Ernest and I had planned on going before we knew that David's T-cells were dropping. Now we wondered how fast the disease might progress. Was it safe for us to leave the United States, even only for two or three weeks? Should we cancel our trip?

We did go to Scotland, but kept in close telephone contact with our home base. The wedding was lovely. My English family was warm, welcoming and grateful that we had come all this way to share in their happiness. Even though I did not tell them about our heartbreak, I felt comforted.

Scotland was more spectacular than I had anticipated. The hills and lochs were abloom with lavender-colored rhododendrons and purple foxgloves. I cried a lot, but recouped some of my strength. By the time we returned home I was in better control of my feelings and felt that I could help my son cope with this mysterious illness.

My inner pain, however, was always there and my eyes misted over constantly. It became increasingly difficult to deal with sad stories. The beggars on the street made me cry, the newspapers with their constant reports of cruelties, massacres, senseless killings, wars and famines, became a burden. I identified with my mother-in-law, who, during her last rather peaceful years, lived with us. "I want happy stories," she used to say, "I want to laugh a bit."

Within weeks after my return from Europe I flew to California. I had not seen David since he got the disastrous T-cell count. David picked me up at the airport and we hugged extra long.

Ever since David had asked me to feel his swollen lymph glands, my unconscious had to contend with the possibility that my son was positive for the AIDS virus. I could not express my fears openly. No matter how terrified and sad I was I could not succumb to grief. I was determined to help David live as full and happy a life as he could. I would not let him glimpse my own panic and despair.

I developed a split personality. Part of me believed that David would make it. Even though I could not even formulate the thought in the privacy of my mind, my other half knew that I might have to help the child to whom I had given life, die. It was a tall order.

Fortunately, David and I shared an immense capability of enjoying life. My son could turn ordinary events into adventures. During that visit David took me to Alan Crouch's birthday party, held in Marin County, along the cliffs overlooking the Golden Gate. The sky was blue, the hills golden. Sailboats filled the sparkling water of the Bay.

David and I joined a group of about 40 men, many paired. I was the only woman present except one. The "boys" wore shorts, T-shirts, hats, caps, jeans—America's standard leisure clothes. At first I was a bit self-conscious, but then I simply enjoyed myself. Where else would I be so special among so many extremely handsome men? Besides, I was consciousness-raising for women and for mothers. Indeed, several people came over to David to tell him that they wished they could bring their mothers to a party like this.

David wanted to show me his office. He introduced me to his boss, and it was as if I was back on parents' day in elementary school to discuss his performance with his teacher. At Gary's house I cooked extra special meals. I explored San Francisco. Most of all I felt comforted looking at my son. He was healthy looking and strong. How could he be fatally ill? My visit drew to a close. I hated to leave. Would David still be all right next time I saw him?

I remembered the way my grandmother used to bless me when I left on a trip. Before boarding the plane I put my hands on David's head garbling the long-forgotten words of the prayer:

May the Lord bless you and keep you
May the Lord lift up His countenance unto you
and grant you peace...

I hoped God would listen to my heart speaking through my imperfect words.

I was not the only member of the family journeying out to California for support. Judy visited and so did Ernest.

It was difficult for Ernest too face his son's fate—what parent can? He fantasized about David being very ill, and returning to his old room in Manhattan and "just in case," he had it equipped with an air-conditioner.

◆   ◆   ◆

I assumed a bi-coastal life-style, visiting David and commuting back to New York where I worked, worried, and looked after my mother. One day I accompanied Judy to her midwives and listened to the twins' heartbeats. "Would they be healthy and normal?" I wondered. Was it AIDS or age that had finally made me lose confidence in the basic goodness of life? One of Judy's twins was breech and the babies would have to be delivered by a Caesarean section. "Another worry," I sighed silently.

The twins were born on August 26, 1987. Within hours of their delivery I saw Ana Teresa Gordon-Loebl and Naomi Rosa Gordon-Loebl, my small claim to immortality. They were small but perfectly healthy. I was overjoyed to have two more people to love, though I knew that love and pain were like the two sides of a coin.

David was ecstatic about his nieces. He visited when they were six weeks old, loving the little girls as if they were the children he knew he would not have.

During that visit David and I took my dog for a long walk in the old cemetery adjoining our apartment house in Manhattan. David was anemic from the AZT, and had trouble walking up hills. During happier times, when his wishes were easily met, he always told his friends, "my mom will come through." Now we both knew that I would do my best to help him face this killer disease. "I think a lot about the Holocaust," he told me, "and that you made it. Perhaps I will make it too."

David's fortitude reassured me. I had witnessed him panic beyond all reason during minor crises, as when a bus driver refused to let him board the bus with his dog, or become hysterical when he had to cope with a standard shift car. Now that it really mattered, I realized he would be brave and determined, and do whatever was necessary to try to save his life.

◆   ◆   ◆

My stress indicators were at their maximum. Sleep often eluded me. I shuddered when the phone rang unexpectedly or flinched when somebody suddenly entered a room. Sometimes I started a sentence and did not finish it. I kept calling David in California, showered him with little presents and hoped that my concern would keep the virus at bay. I was very lonely.

There was nobody with whom I could talk about my heartache. I had to be brave with David. Judy was so sad about the possibility of losing her brother that I did not want to burden her with my fear. My husband could not bear my anguish. I have always hated being pitied. I usually am the strong one, and rarely find it necessary to confide in my friends.

To bolster myself I recalled the strength of other women. The ones who had watched their sons go off to war; those who encouraged their children to leave for America before there were fast ships and planes; the mothers who watched their children die of cancer or in car accidents. None of that helped. It occurred to me that there must be other mothers living in the shadow of the AIDS virus. But where were they? Perhaps the gay community, which by then had vigorously responded to the AIDS crisis, might have a support group for someone like me. Because even something as non-committal as a phone call meant that my dread was grounded in reality, it took fortitude to dial the number of the Gay Men's Health Crisis. I was referred to Frank Donnelly, the co-facilitator of group that met weekly in Greenwich Village. Frank asked me how old David was. "Thirty-one," I answered. "You'll fit right in," Frank said sadly. It seemed that I had found some buddies.

3

THE MOTHERS GROUP

It had taken me so long to find people with whom to share my plight that I went to the Mothers' group every Tuesday when I was in town. Age-wise my new friends ranged from their early forties to their late seventies. Since in 1987 AIDS affected mostly gay men, the women who met in the Living Room were already battle-scarred. Most of us had had a hard time accepting our sons' homosexuality. After we did we faced a society that condemned homosexuality and held mothers responsible for their children's life-style. Now many people felt that gays themselves were responsible for this new plague.

Standing by an HIV-infected child required determination. The mothers of my group were telling the world: "My son is gay. I love my son. He is suffering from a dreadful, deadly disease. I am sharing his plight."

Fran Hermann had been living in California with a new partner when her son called from New York announcing that he had AIDS. Fran came for a brief visit. Eric, however, needed round the clock care, and she stayed. By the time it was all over she had lost both her son and her lover.

Fran had missed people with whom to share her ordeal. A social worker by training, she felt that "during a crisis women usually provide the emotional strength for the entire family—husbands, children, their own aging parents—and never get a chance to express their own fears and needs." To help others to cope better, she had founded the support group

The Mothers Group filled an obvious need. A single woman had shown up at the initial meeting in 1986. Six months later I was the 43rd mother to avail herself of its warmth and wisdom. During its eight-year long existence the group welcomed 350 women.

I hated the Mothers' Group and I loved it. Through attending it I openly confronted the realities of this puzzling disease once a week. I identified with the misery and helplessness of the others. Their stories fuelled my fear, and on Tuesday nights sleep eluded me even more consistently than on other nights. Yet, the brave part of my personality was buoyed by what I witnessed. If the other women managed to live with and through AIDS, I could too.

The group also kindled hope. Sophisticated new drugs like AZT seemed to stem the AIDS virus. There was talk about effective vaccines and there were scores of alternate treatments. I felt that provided he remained healthy, David might beat the odds. In 1987, however, there was no way of predicting how long it would take for anyone to develop overt AIDS.

Most weeks there were new mothers. Most had gay sons. Most were middle class. Some came regularly, others suddenly showed up one evening, heartbroken, sharing their helplessness. Some had always supported their gay children; others had not known that their sons were gay. Now they had to confront their child's homosexuality and face his imminent death.

We all felt guilty and responsible. Were we to blame for our son's homosexuality and consequently his disease? Was it true that gay sons had domineering mothers and passive fathers?

One evening, when one of us again embarked on this well worn theme, Frank Donnelly recalled how difficult it had been for him, during the 1940's, to grow up Catholic and gay, in a small, ultra-conservative New Jersey town. Frank remembered his mother's love and protection. He never came out to her, though he was convinced that her love shielded him from a distant, abusive father and a hostile world. Frank's tale reminded me of Dan Rosenblatt, who also never told his mom about his homosexuality.

"Fathers often are threatened by their sons' homosexuality," Frank said. "It may echo their doubts about their own sexual orientation or masculinity. My own father simply was not good at fixing cars or playing ball, which is how society defined masculinity in the 1950's. Homosexuality is inborn," Frank continued. "In my own family there are uncles and nieces who are openly gay, and a number of nuns and priests who took refuge in the Church."

◆   ◆   ◆

I had joined the Mothers' group the week Rick Dixon died, and I had not shared his mother's final ordeal. During that first meeting Deane talked about the candles, flowers, and food she was getting for her son's memorial. Thereafter she planned to take the ferry to Fire Island and scattered Rick's ashes in the ocean. "How could this woman do all that? I wondered in disbelief.

Later, when Deane had become a friend, she told me her family's story.

Her marriage to Paul had always been stormy, especially after Deane became an over-conscientious kindergarten teacher. Paul was bossy and possessive, and resented his wife's devotion to her work. One day he simply locked Deane out of the house. As she recalled, "For one reason or another I could never move back in." Her children, 17-year-old Gretel and 12-year-old Rick, stayed with their father. Actually Rick, who was very close to Deane, had expected his mother to come and fetch him, but she failed to understand his need.

When Rick was in high school he ran away from home. His parents, by now divorced, consulted the school's guidance counselor, who recommended that Rick be sent to a psychotherapist.

"Paul and I believed that the therapist would solve Rick's problems," Dean remembered. "Rick calmed down, graduated from high school and went off to college."

Since Rick had always dated girls, Deane did not suspected that he was gay, but once when she went to visit him in college she found him in bed with another man. Deane was shocked and Rick mortified that his mother had discovered his secret.

"I believed all that stuff about the bossy mother and the weak father," Deane recalled "and I felt guilty." Eventually she got used to the idea of Rick being gay. "After I met my son's kind, smart and handsome friends I made peace with myself. I concluded that the stereotypical picture of a 'queer' was hogwash. By the time Rick got AIDS I was past all that gay stuff."

Rick probably was infected with the HIV virus in 1978, long before there was any talk of AIDS. In June of that year he developed flu-like symptoms, swollen glands, and lost a great deal of weight. The brief illness was forgotten. Six years later, Rick developed Kaposi sarcoma (KS) and was diagnosed with AIDS.

"Rick told me right away that he had AIDS. I started to cry, and simply could not stop." He did not share his news with either his father or his sister, who was a Seventh Day Adventist. He swore his mother to secrecy.

"From the very beginning I felt that Rick was going to die," Deane recalled, "but I never let him know. I clung to straws; one was a rumor that people who had KS lasted longer."

Telling others about one's HIV status is like jumping off a cliff blindfolded. I remember David agonizing each time he had to tell someone new: a boss, a date, or even a beloved, long-time friend, that he was a carrier. How would the news be received? How many doors would now be closed? How would he now appear to others? Fifty years ago cancer carried a similar stigma, and people rarely revealed their diagnosis. This additional burden is superfluous. Even back then, HIV carriers continued to lead normal, productive lives and made extraordinary contributions to humanity.

Ostracism, however, is only one reason for not telling. None of us can face our own mortality. For those infected as well as for their partners, it is easier to forget about the disease as long as it is secret. Even though David never asked me to keep his HIV status hidden, I was reluctant to share my heartache with others. Not discussing the most important aspect of my life with my close friends, however, increased my isolation.

Rick's unwillingness to tell even his nuclear family that he was fatally ill saddled Deane with an additional burden.

"It was a terrible time." Deane recalled. "I was still teaching in Long Island. I was a true workaholic. I had a history of never being absent. Then suddenly I became totally enmeshed in my son's illness of which I was not allowed to talk."

Rick, like every ailing child, regardless of age, wanted his mother. On some level, all us mothers were dealing with loving, charming, selfish, rude, and irresponsible overgrown infants.

Rick was more fortunate than others. Patrick Hennessy, his physician, managed to have him participate in some of the early treatment studies at the National Institutes of Health (NIH) in Bethesda, MD. Even though some of the nurses at our national hospital were homophobic, and felt that "AIDS was what gays deserved," Rick liked being in Maryland.

After his discharge he moved back to his apartment in New York. His disease progressed rapidly. He developed AIDS dementia and was incapable of managing a large sum of money awarded to him for a car accident. By 1986 he was in and out of different hospitals, including the NIH, Bellevue's psychiatric ward, and New York Hospital.

"I still lived on Long Island, near my job," Deane recalled, "but I spent more and more time in the city with Rick. Going back and forth was just too much, and I finally quit teaching. I could not do two job anymore."

"It was not easy to care for Rick. Often I felt like committing suicide. I did discuss his illness with some of my friends, and then I found the Mothers' Group." Deane became a faithful attendant. In between meetings she snuck out of Rick's apartment, went to a public phone and called one of the other mothers. "I would not have survived Rick's last months without the Mothers' Group."

Even after Rick died, Deane kept coming to the Tuesday meetings, becoming the group's self-appointed secretary and historian. She kept our records with the same diligence with which she had managed her kindergarten classes. Each new mother received a handwritten list with every group member's phone number.

Assuring everyone that she did not sleep at night, she encouraged us to call her anytime we needed to. Deane never forgot any of the women who came to seek support, no matter how fleetingly, and contributed to the group's smooth running and survival.

◆   ◆   ◆

In October 1987, a few months after I joined the Mothers' group, my phone rang. David was calling from Kaiser Permanente Hospital in Oakland. He had developed severe anemia from the AZT, and required a blood transfusion. He was alone in the hospital, though eventually Brian, one of his roommates, showed up with a pizza. How I wished that I were in San Francisco.

During the early years of the AIDS epidemic everybody thought that the virus killed quickly, within a matter of two years or less. Ernest and I decided that I would spend extended periods of time in California, even though I was the principal caregiver of my aging, increasingly helpless mother, and the double rent and other expenses would strain our finances.

David seemed to welcome such support. One day he called and teasingly asked whether I knew what happens to mothers whose sons have gotten respectable jobs? I said that I had no idea. "They get taken to Hawaii," he told me. David had booked a Kauai vacation for the two of us.

He met me at the San Francisco airport. His blue eyes were beaming, but he was clearly worried.

"How do I look?" he asked anxiously. I had to admit that he was kind of pale. We struggled with my over-heavy suitcase. "I am no longer in great shape," he said.

I accompanied David to his next appointment with Dr. Marks. I had not gone with my son to the doctor since he was a child. From now on, whenever I was in California, this became part of the routine. I knew that my presence reduced David's anxiety and that my medical knowledge impressed doctors. Even without these advantages, I knew that physicians usually try a little harder when an additional person is present.

In 1987 the recommended dose of AZT was so high that it often caused severe anemia. Moreover, the long-term effectiveness of AZT was unknown. Marks felt that if David continued with the AZT he would require periodic blood transfusions. This in itself was risky. To improve the quality of David's life, Marks advised discontinuing AZT. The final decision, however, was up too David. It was a difficult choice, since AZT was the only available anti-AIDS drug. In the end, David opted to get off AZT.

My medical reporter eyes could see that AIDS was going to change the practice of medicine. The disease was so novel, and so deadly, and doctors knew so little about its treatment, that they eagerly shared the decision-making process with their patients.

Days after he stopped AZT David started to feel better, but he had a long way to go to recapture his strength. We left on Thanksgiving Day. To my son's delight, we were greeted with a traditional lei of flowers. We picked up our car, found our hotel and at David's insistence went to the Sheraton for a traditional Thanksgiving feast.

David's insistence on having it all reminded me of when he was one year old. To make sure that he would not miss anything important, he would wake up each morning long before the rest of the family. I fished him out of his crib before he woke Judy, Ernest or Grandma, and for an hour he was all mine and I was all his.

We spent five glorious days on Kauai. We did not know what the future held, but we loved the present. We slithered in the mud beneath the towering cliffs of the Napali coast, bathed on hidden beaches, ate with the locals at a noodle shop and lived it up at a fancy restaurant. One day we took a helicopter and had an air-view of Kauwaiaii's spectacular cliffs and jagged mountains peaks. The copter buzzed Waimea canyon, inhabited by the Hawaiian ancestors, and flew over Hanalee, the home of Puff, the magic dragon. The earth was a dangerous place, but oh, how much fun it could be.

I wanted to hover over David like a mother hen. I could "see" the bacteria teeming in the potato salad or congregating on the sushi. Did he get enough sleep? Was he getting too much sun? I knew, however, that David did not need a nurse, but rather my absolute conviction that he would beat AIDS. Indeed, as I listened to his laugh, watched his skin tan, and noticed that he could climb hills without getting short of breath, I willed myself to think that AIDS was a nightmare that would vanish at dawn.

When we returned to San Francisco I looked for an apartment. Within the week I had rented an unfurnished one bedroom on Chetwood Street, around the corner from Gary's house on Santa Clara Avenue. I furnished the place with much pleasure. I rented and borrowed furniture, bought stuff at garage sales and in thrift shops. David handed me a large box. It held a weird assemblage of goods, some from Alan and David's Boston household, some dating from my parents' home in Germany, some discards from our summer cottage in Maine. I was surprised and sad to unpack this assorted junk, kept for odd, sentimental reasons. Plants, posters and photos of my new granddaughters completed the interior decoration. It was the first time in my life that I made a nest just for myself alone, and I enjoyed it.

I fell in love with California—the friendly people, the weather, the fresh fruits and vegetables, the easy lifestyle. I had brought my computer and had enough work to keep me busy during the day. Writing enabled me to handle the uncertain, unnerving times.

Except for Bonnie Remsberg and Rick Bode—two fellow writers who had just relocated 30 miles down the coast—I had no friends of my own. I did not mind. I am a loner at heart. My own vulnerability made me cautious of forming new friendships. David's friends were glad of my mothering presence and adopted me with open arms.

◆　　　◆　　　◆

I missed my Mothers and hastily searched for a replacement. A suitable group met weekly at a Baptist Church in Oakland, within walking distance of my abode. The group was small, unstructured and relaxed. Participants included mothers, fathers and friends of patients with AIDS or AIDS-Related Complex (ARC for short), then considered an earlier, milder stage of AIDS. Group sessions often started with extensive small talk, but after a while we shared the trials and small victories of the past week. The stories in Oakland were just as wrenching as those in New York.

Just then Matty, a gay single father and the sports coach of a local high school, took over as co-facilitator. On his first evening the members of the group told their stories. Phyllis Jones and her husband, Mark, began.

This was a second marriage for both Phyllis and Mark. Between them they had six children, and nine grandchildren. Holidays in the Jones' house had been very happy affairs, with 22 at the table for Thanksgiving and even more for Christmas dinner.

Phyllis recalled: "I was a real Christmas junkie, the tree, the gifts, the lights, the food, the candy, the stockings, the whole bit." That's how things were an eternity ago—last year.

In June, Mark's son, Tom, told Phyllis, who described herself as the "Dear Abby" of her large family, that he had AIDS. He warned her not to tell the rest of the family yet. But when Mark came home that night, he saw that Phyllis had been crying. It did not take him long to discover the reason, and he too cried.

Two months later Tom had to be hospitalized, and after discharge he came to stay with Phyllis and Mark.

Phyllis learned as much about AIDS as she could from books, pamphlets and videotapes published by the San Francisco AIDS Foundation, the Surgeon General, and the National Institutes of Health. She knew that the disease was not transmitted by casual social contact. Her children and stepchildren believed otherwise. Phyllis begged them to read some of the literature she had collected or at least view the videotape. The children simply refused to visit while Tom was home. Even after he had gotten better and returned to his own house, some hundred miles down the coast, they shunned Phyllis' and Mark's house. Tom started to take AZT and did well, but his brothers and sisters still would not have anything to do with him.

All that was in August. The holidays came, and Tom's siblings did not relent. There was no Thanksgiving turkey, and no Christmas dinner. A few of the family members dropped in Christmas morning, but the grandchildren were not allowed to run around the house as they once did. "Their parents made them sit in the living room," Phyllis told us, in a voice that she had trouble controlling. "They were not even permitted to have a piece of Christmas candy.

"How am I going to explain to my grandchildren that I love them more than ever; that none of this is my doing!"

Listening to Phyllis and Mark made me think of my own sweet daughter, who was standing by her brother and was letting him enjoy her children.

◆　　　◆　　　◆

David told me one day: "We'll always remember that we had this time together." Indeed, that Oakland winter was special. I missed my husband and my new grandchildren in New York. I regretted neglecting my mother, but I loved being on my own, and felt that it was important to share my son's joys and frustrations.

There were many of the latter. As always, David loved and hated with passion. By now he disliked his job at AT&T. He hated his doctor, Stephen Marks, whose AIDS therapy was too conservative. He minded living at Gary's, still missed Jeff, and was scared of AIDS.

Once the gay community had acknowledged AIDS, it fought the disease with intelligence and immense compassion. Within a very short time major AIDS organizations sprang to life: GMHC, AMFAR, PWAC, SFAF, Project Inform and a whole alphabet soup of others. The main thrust of these organizations differed. Some stressed advocacy, others emphasized research or the dissemination of medical information, others provided services. One organization, PAWS, short for Pets Are Wonderful Support, saw to it that patients were able to hang on to their dogs and cats.

I was David's medical sleuth. I read every relevant lay and scientific report about AIDS and AIDS drugs, attended every press conference. I told my science writing colleagues that my son was HIV positive in the hope that they would let me know when something new was on the horizon. I was well equipped. Ironically, my first book, *Fighting the Unseen,* had dealt with the discovery of viruses and vaccines. The first virus had been discovered only in 1898. Ninety years later these tiny infectious agents were still causing havoc.

When in San Francisco, I attended the monthly health forums organized by Project Inform, an AIDS organization that assembled, evaluated and disseminated any available medical information. Looking at the audience—vigorous men in their thirties, forties and fifties, all infected with the deadly virus—made me sick. These men were not going to go quietly. They were determined and brave. Where were the freaks, the sissies, the wimps, the flakes, those stereotypes many straight people equate with being homosexual?

The AIDS epidemic was the first time in history that those threatened by a disease took an active part in shaping its treatment. AIDS patients battled the government, the FDA, and their doctors. Pentamidine was seldom used before the advent of PCP, the fatal AIDS-related pneumonia. A preliminary study showed that the prophylactic use of aerosol pentamidine dramatically decreased the incidence of PCP. Even before the study was completed, the gay community insisted that the prophylactic use of pentamadine become standard treatment,

The cost of AZT was sky high. In 1987 ACT-UP, a gay activist group, marched into the New York Stock Exchange, strewing fake dollar bills all over the place. For the first time ever, the Exchange had to be closed, and eventually Burroughs-Welcome, the manufacturer of AZT, agreed to drop the price of the drug.

Even though these were small victories, I admired the gay community's determination. Self-pity was disdained. Referring to anyone infected by the HIV-virus as a victim was now a faux pas, tantamount to calling an African-American a "nigger." It was hard for the wounded-well, like me, not to cry when seeing emaciated, Kaposi-ridden, pale, chemo-therapied, bent-over people half my age, but these were the rules of the game.

◆   ◆   ◆

I returned to New York in February, 1988, to help my mother celebrate her 86th birthday. I kept the Oakland apartment, planning to come back in the spring. While I was gone my quarters were used by Judy, John, the twins, Ernest and Michael Leak—one of David's Provincetown friends.

I remember one painful incident that occurred during my absence. Deane wrote a postcard reporting that five of the Mothers, Arlene, Rae, Florence, and the two Nancys, had lost their children: David intercepted the card and sent it on to New York with a note affirming his determination to live:

Hi my Mom!

I am pretty happy these days, especially since I now have my, rather our, little apartment back! I got the check—thanks so much.—

The postcard you got is sort of depressing—sorry!! Don't worry—I'm not going to add my name to that unfortunate list!!

Tonight is pentamadine, tomorrow Margie [his psychotherapist] and FRIDAY my birthday! (YAY!) I'm not sure what I'll do yet. Probably arrange a dinner for myself with Alan (Crouch) and a few others.

Unofficially I found out my ranking (and raise for next year: # 4 and $ 2500 (7.5 %) that's not too bad!!

Lots and Lots of Love

David

I was back in Oakland for my birthday on May 14th, which that year fell on a Saturday. That morning David came with flowers, a chocolate cake, a check for $200 and a card that said, *"I want you to know how much I appreciate what you are doing for me."*

One day I got a call from Anne Williams, whose son, Brian, was a friend of David's. She was writing a master's thesis on mothers' reactions to their children's homosexuality. During the interview I had not been quite candid about how painful it had been, in the dim past, to reconcile myself to David's sexual orientation.

My caution had been well founded. Carelessly, Anne lent her thesis to her son, who lent it to David, who told me that he recognized who I was because I was the only European mother among those discussed. He had no other comments.

I had told Anne about David's HIV status and she was most sympathetic. She was convinced that her Brian was OK. Three years later, Brian developed AIDS-related leukemia.

Gradually Judy and I started to relax a bit about David's state of health. We both felt that we would not lose him overnight. When David finally moved from his room in Gary's house to a spectacular apartment in San Francisco, I reluctantly dismantled my Oakland apartment because it was too distant from my son's new abode. For the time being I knew that he did not need a mother hovering close by, and figured that I would arrange for temporary quarters as needed.

Ernest came out and to help me pack and help David move to 902 Haight Street. The three of us had a good time, and then the older Loebls returned to New York.

4

"GIVE ME THE STRENGTH"

Disasters alter resolves. One long-standing resolve of mine had been not to hang on to my grown children. By the time Judy and David went off to college I was engrossed in my own career. AIDS catapulted me back right into the center of David's life. My concern with his health and happiness were always uppermost in my mind, and the many other aspects of my life paled by comparison. I was as involved with him as I'd been when he was an infant, except that now he was a grown man. David, for his part became very dependent on me. He felt more secure when I was around.

It was as if the umbilical cord had grown back. Often, when I called California, David said, "I was just thinking about you." To me this was not surprising. David was constantly in my thoughts; it was as if thinking about him kept the disease at bay. Whenever I realized that he had escaped from my consciousness for a few hours, my anxiety surged with renewed vigor.

I witnessed similar intense bonding between other mothers and their stricken children. Whether we were with them or not, concern about their health governed our lives.

Major crises create emotional mine fields. I was neglecting my husband, my daughter and my friends. Still, my marriage was solid enough to withstand the assault, and Judy was so close to her brother that she did not seem to mind. In my Mothers' Group, however, I saw that devotion to an HIV-infected child often shattered other long-standing commitments.

Nothing, however, is simple. I worried that my unwavering support prevented my son from finding a new partner. On the other hand my ready availability probably did not matter. David was extremely cautious about forming new bonds. He had been so deeply hurt when he lost Jeff, and was so terrified by his HIV status, that he seemed unable to fall in love.

David was not the only HIV-positive man to have such problems. In the gay community, AIDS permeated all relationships. The HIV-negative men felt guilty about being healthy. Some HIV-positive guys lied about or denied their status and infected new partners. In time three groups emerged, each keeping mostly to itself. The sero-negatives were reluctant to become involved with those positive for the HIV virus. The infected-well did not want to be burdened with anyone further along the road to full-blown AIDS. Those suffering from overt AIDS usually did not have the strength to become romantically involved.

These schisms were just another aspect of the stress of living in the time of AIDS. I knew from David the hassle of having to discuss his HIV status with new acquaintances. Fortunately, he had a solid core of friends and no trouble finding dates.

In retrospect, it surprises me how much happiness I experienced being there for David. I did not want to crowd him or act as if I was waiting for him to become sick. So I usually visited for a few weeks three or even four times a year. Even then I often did not stay with him, and he too preferred me to be on my own.

As I was searching for quarters in San Francisco, I discovered Family Link, an AIDS hostel located a few blocks from David's new digs on Haight Street. The lodging was the brainchild of Sister Ruth Hall, a nun of the order of Saint Francis, and of Ray Cope, her associate. Sister Ruth's convent had kept a guest room used by visiting family members. When AIDS struck, this single room could not accommodate the many who came to see those living with, or dying from the disease. Sister Ruth and Ray managed to rent several apartments with rooms for those who were in San Francisco on "AIDS business." Now Family Link was able to provide creature comforts, transportation to and from the airport, immense compassion, and addresses for essential services. Sister Ruth and Ray were always ready to listen, console and advise.

In spite of all that goodness, I was unhappy at Family Link. Most of the other guests came to bid a last farewell to a son or a brother, or to attend funerals. Their anguish, their rage, their regret of not having known, their remorse at not having made peace with their sons' homosexuality, their pain at outliving their children, and sometimes their eagerness at inheriting their earthly belongings were stifling. Since I was in California to help David vanquish the virus I could not afford to be overwhelmed by second-hand grief. My son was well and I came to buoy up his spirit.

Ernest felt differently about Family Link. Since he did not have a support group, the hostel provided him with the strength to deal with his sometimes cantankerous son. He even bonded with a boot-wearing father from Texas, who was there to make peace with the son who had fallen so far from the family tree.

I always tried to shield David from AIDS' deadly outcome, and avoided having him visit me at Family Link. I cleansed my own mind in the few blocks that separated Family Link from David's spectacular apartment on Haight Street.

When I got there I had to a climb nearly eighty steps to reach the renovated duplex that Keith Potter, a promising commercial artist, and David had rented in an old Victorian house. The ascent was well worth it. From one of the enormous living room windows one could see the sun rise over the Bay, from another one glimpsed the gnarled pines of Buena Vista Park.

"Have you ever seen something that beautiful?" David asked me when I first got there.

The apartment was ideal for parties. I usually visited in February for David's birthday and helped him organize a mammoth celebration. I find cooking therapeutic, and prepared enough food to feed an army. It was never wasted. David's friends loved home-cooked meals. Most of them had struggled in "coming out," and many were still at odds with their parents. A mother who went all out to support her son was a rarity. Everybody felt defeated by "the plague" and loved being mothered. The "boys" felt comfortable with me there, and told off-color in-jokes. They seemed amazed that my presence did not embarrass them. I too was surprised. What had happened to the woman who could not face her son being gay?

David's phone rang constantly with calls from his many friends. There were his "Seven Sisters," a group of male friends who often vacationed together; old friends from the Boston days and Provincetown; newer ones from business school and AT&T. David had straight friends and, women friends, and was such fun to party with that he was much in demand as an escort. Then there was his special Halloween crowd. For months before this, the holiest of all gay holidays, they discussed what they would be: Gays in the Military, bathing beauties, Rockettes, Josephine Baker…Then they sewed the drag costumes, made hats, and wigs and size nine high-heels. The annual madness concluded with the group usually winning first prize at a Halloween ball.

Two of David's friends, Dave Nelson and Frank Hawkins, were also infected with the AIDS virus. This made their relationship with my son particularly close. Each of these men handled his burden differently. Dave Nelson withdrew within himself when the talk turned to AIDS. David Loebl explored every hopeful treatment alternative. Frank defied the virus by becoming a champion swimmer. At parties no one could have guessed that these three had a care in the world. David and Frank were natural comedians. When they embarked on one of their favorite routines, imitating Bette Mittler or Ronald Reagan, everybody laughed until they hurt.

Because the theater was one of David's avocations, he decided to exploit his acting talent. He enrolled in a class taught by Rick Mason. Eventually Rick produced a play, entitled The Gays of our Lives, which got respectable reviews in the gay press.

All this activity was one indication of the schizophrenic nature of David's life. As I watched my son's fingers constantly caress the swollen lymph glands in his neck, I knew that he never forgot about his HIV status. Those close to David were aware of his short fuse. The slightest provocation or mishap, such as the upstairs neighbor complaining about his loud radio, parking tickets, or hassles with insurance companies, could trigger a hysterical outburst on David's part. He had occasional altercations with everyone he loved.

When I was with him I tried to be on my best behavior, keeping his abode as clean and orderly as I could. Sometimes he still got very angry. I tried not to take it personally. Often he would write me a little note afterwards apologizing. Nevertheless, my visits reassured both of us. How could anything be wrong with my fun-loving, if angry son? He too felt reassured. Aren't mothers always capable of protecting their young?

I had a harder time coping with AIDS in New York. Feeling that I lived on the rim of an active volcano, betwixt earthquakes, or on the fringe of a tornado, I was constantly searching for crutches, safety belts, and crash helmets.

I am a secular Jew, and always felt uncomfortable with organized religion. I never got over the childish notion of a well-meaning, white-bearded God, who was there to take care of me. I was unfamiliar with rituals, couldn't read Hebrew, and felt out of place in a synagogue. But my involvement with AIDS was such, that when Congregation B'nai Jeshurun, on Manhattan's Upper West Side, held an AIDS Seder, Ernest and I went. I was pleased that, though the Bible considers homosexuality a major transgression, the two rabbis, Marshall Meyer and Roland Matalon, courageously accepted openly gay parishioners.

I started to attend Sabbath Services at the temple. I left my home early Saturday morning, often before my husband was up, to spent time with myself. I entered the lavish, Moorish-inspired sanctuary. Each week I took the same seat, half way down the left aisle. My mind rattled with everyday concerns: the coat that needed to go to the cleaners, the weekly shopping, or my Mom's new caretaker. Slowly the organ music, the extraordinary voices of Marshall and Roli and of the cantor, the rhythmic cadence of the prayers calmed my overactive brain.

I bonded with generations of Jews—my grandparents, their parents, my parents. I felt their strength. I knew many had faltered, some lived good lives, some had perished during the Holocaust, yet they all had kept the faith. Their blood flowed in my veins. I owed them my compassion, my good judgment, my positive attitude, my determination. Most of all I owed them the ability to do the right thing whenever humanly possible.

My life had never been easy. First there were the Nazis in Germany, quarreling parents, uprooting, the Holocaust, more uprooting. Yet I had always enjoyed the battle and the challenge. It was as if I told the world: "You'll see, I am going to make it." And I had made it. I had a husband, children, a country, a profession, friends and creature comforts.

Fate had kept its worst card for last—the AIDS epidemic that threatened my child. I did not know whether I would come through it. I knew that I would do my best: for David, for Judy, for Ernest, for my grandchildren, for myself, for all the Jews who shielded that tiny flame while holocausts and typhoons raged around them.

After the service at B'nai Jeshurun, I spent the afternoon with my Mom, David's beloved Omi. I was more gracious than usual as I prepared lunch, played Scrabble, looked at her poor old wrinkled face and watched in horror as her mind slowly clouded over.

◆ ◆ ◆

David had now entrusted his health to Dr. Marcus Conant. During the two decades preceding AIDS, Conant had been a successful dermatologist at the University of California Medical School. He was smart, good looking, witty and gay. Speaking with the drawl of his native South, Conant never tired telling how he had witnessed homosexuals creeping out of their closets, opening gay bars and hanging rainbow-colored flags from their windows. In 1981 Conant and a few other dermatologists had been alarmed by the outbreak of Kaposi sarcoma among gay men. This "gay cancer" indeed had proved to be one of the hallmarks of AIDS.

Rapidly, Conant moved to the forefront of AIDS treatment. In the spring of 1988, when David became his patient, Conant still saw him personally. He was reassuring and personable. Later, physicians' assistants provided the routine care, while Conant became more and more absorbed in AIDS research and politics. We felt that this was to our advantage, since Conant had ready access to all the new AIDS drugs. When I told my Mothers' Group that David was Conant's patient, my friends were reassuring. "He is one of the best," Deane said.

AIDS was a heavy burden for the medical profession, both physically and emotionally. Doctors and nurses identified with their young patients. These men's inevitable deaths left their health care providers frustrated and defeated. Eventually some caregivers became callous, others burnt out, while others still were able to deliver excellent, compassionate care for as long as required. Nevertheless, because of AIDS' relentless progression, most patients ended up resenting their powerless healers.

None of these tensions surfaced in Conant's elegant waiting room, decorated by one of David's recent "dates." Conant's patients were young, healthy-looking men. The tasteful space reminded me of the antechambers of pre-World War II consulates where "the damned" hoped for a visa allowing them to escape from Hitler's inferno. The question "who shall live and who shall die," asked during the Yom Kippur services, kept echoing in my head.

After David's physical was over, I joined him and Tina Clark or Marc Illeman in the examining room. David was holding his own, one or the other of these physician's assistants assured us. His "numbers" (results of the blood tests) were good. New drugs were in the pipeline. We were eager to believe the cheerful news, and the monthly ordeal over, returned to San Francisco's sunny streets, thinking of how we were to spend the evening.

Actually, David's numbers were not all that good. He had been off AZT for a number of years, but when his T-cells dropped below the magic 200, he resumed taking the antiviral. Tests had shown that AZT was effective at lower doses, which David was able to tolerate. He also had to resume prophylactic aerosol pentamidine treatments. Once a month for one hour, David had to inhale the drug from an aerosol dispenser. I sometimes went to keep him company.

I got to know Dr. Conant rather well, not only in San Francisco, but also during various press conferences and science writers' meetings at which he was a featured speaker. I was impressed by his insight and knowledge. Conant realized that traditional medicine, with the authoritarian physician and the obedient patient, would not work for AIDS. To help the gay community participate in their own care, he convened a monthly town meeting at which he discussed the latest developments in AIDS therapy and research. Like the Project Inform symposia, the meetings were packed with healthy looking men. Their questions indicated their AIDS expertise; their laughter, an affirmation of their courage and determination to survive.

At first David went to the meetings, taking extensive notes. Eventually the pictures of end-stage AIDS patients, which Conant routinely projected, frightened him. Whenever I could, I went in his stead. At these town meetings Conant summarized the information presented at the annual World AIDS conferences. It became apparent that the HIV virus survived because it could change its genetic makeup so as to elude old and new drugs. Conant's hopes centered on D4T, a drug that prevented the virus from attaching to susceptible white blood cells. He told his patients to "hang on" for two years until the new drug became available.

Whenever conventional medicine is stymied, unproven remedies and alternative therapies flourish. Throughout history some folk remedies have proved effective and life saving. Two hundred years earlier, Edward Jenner, practicing in rural England, had listened to a milkmaid and came up with a vaccine that eradicated smallpox, a viral disease as devastating as AIDS. Digitalis, a compound isolated from the foxglove plant, assisted failing hearts, and aspirin-like drugs stilled fever and alleviated rheumatism long before anyone understood why.

Unfortunately, most folk remedies, including copper bracelets and some supposed vitamins, are useless, expensive, and occasionally harmful. Moreover, their employ may delay the use of more effective medication. There was, however, no effective AIDS therapy, and all patients, including my son, felt that they could not neglect any promising therapy. I supported his efforts, provided he kept Conant informed.

Some of these alternate forms of therapy were trucked in from Mexico, others were available through various specialized Buyer's Clubs, and others still were almost mainstream. David had acupuncture treatments. His Chinese herbalist supplied him with forty pills a day, to the tune of $150 a month. He took a whole slew of vitamins. I was skeptical about the value of some of these measures, but withheld comment, lest I negate the beneficial psychological effects they might have. When in town, I picked up whatever he needed at the herbalist and the buyers club. Each new treatment provided us with a high. It was going to lick the virus!

I subscribed to truly experimental therapies, hoping that indeed they would save my child. In 1985 an Israeli scientist "discovered" that lipids (fats) derived from egg yolk were effective. The rationale behind this remedy was that the lipids coated the white blood cells, thereby preventing the HIV virus from gaining access. The lipids, mashed with fruit, had to be taken on an empty stomach. For a year or two David faithfully swallowed the egg lipids, until they too were proven ineffective.

Dextran sulfate emerged in 1988. *AIDS Treatment News* and other respectable publications touted its "miraculous effects." Even Conant discussed the drug at his town meetings. This old-fashioned anti-coagulant medication was unavailable in the United States, but widely used in Japan. After a few false starts, I unearthed Hiroko Murata, a Japanese pen pal of my 65-year old cousin Claude. I wrote Hiroko, now married to a physician, a letter that smacks of guerrilla tactics:

July 2, 1988

Dear Hiroko—if I may call you that.

I am Claude Bamberger's first cousin, and I have known about you from the time you were in high school and started corresponding with him…He always spoke very fondly of you. Feeling that I know you, emboldens me to ask you for a big favor.

My son David is suffering from ARC—AIDS Related Complex. As you may know, Dextran Sulfate, which can be bought without prescription in Japan, is currently believed to be a rather effective anti-viral agent…

Within less than two weeks Hiroko sent David a three months' supply of dextran sulfate. David was proud of our resourcefulness in battling the plague. Hiroko became our faithful friend, sending dextran sulfate and little presents for as long as we needed the drug. Unfortunately that drug too proved ineffective. It, however, had been important to try, and while we believed in dextran sulfate, it may very well have had magical power.

When the dextran sulfate bubble burst we fortunately had more solid ground for optimism. In 1990 AZT was no longer the only available AIDS medication. The pharmaceutical industry had developed two other antivirals drugs: DDI and DDC. Conant had access, and David was enrolled in an experimental study. Alternate weeks he took different combinations of these drugs. At his town meetings Conant showed why this treatment might work. We were optimistic. After all, drug combinations had represented a breakthrough in cancer therapy.

Magic is an important aspect of medical care. I had always laughed at my mother's many superstitions: black cats, spilling salt, not washing clothes between Christmas and New Year's, not walking under a ladder. Now I subscribed to many of these. I rejoiced in any good omen. Even when I was not with David, I never touched a glass of wine without toasting his health. When with David, my favorite toast was: "may you bury me." I am a conscious Jew, yet I seldom passed a church without thinking of the Virgin Mary and telling her that she could not "possibly do this to me."

I will forever be grateful that David shared his HIV status with me from the very beginning. I pity mothers who only discover their children's secret during the late stages of the disease. Their agony might be short, but they do not have time to resolve old conflicts or to become familiar with a tragedy that alters the very essence of their lives.

Nevertheless it is difficult to be one's child's care partner. I listened very carefully to David, always walking a thin line between being helpful and being overprotective, being supportive and showing pity, recognizing the seriousness of the situation and projecting doom.

I wanted to be there all the time, yet I did not want to be a burden. Part of me waited for David to become sick and die, while another part refused to acknowledge the precariousness of the situation.

AIDS violated the usual generational contract. Wasn't my grown child supposed to care for me, not me for him? I wanted to scream. I wanted to tell David how scared I was. Instead I had to offer endless reassurance: "Yes," I had to say over and over again, "you are healthy, now and a cure will be available long before you will need it."

Fortunately, I too heard my reassuring words, and in the process of convincing him, often managed to alleviate my own fears.

Because we felt, despite our overt confidence, that our time together might be limited, we made ordinary life extraordinary. Every meal I cooked for David was special. Before I returned to New York, I always filled David's freezer with home-cooked food so that my care surrounded him when I was 3000 miles away.

Luckily during the 1990s one of my books paid handsome royalties, so I could indulge David. His childlike enthusiasm turned every outing into an adventure. We visited wineries and ate fancy meals in Napa. We wallowed in mud baths in Calistoga. We "sat" in a Buddhist Temple and tried to meditate. David avidly read restaurant reviews, and when I visited we tried promising eating establishments. We flew to Los Angeles to see *Phantom of the Opera,* for which David had gotten house seats. In Los Angeles we shopped for clothes. Every woman should have a gay son to go shopping with. Even years later, I feel special when I wear one of our purchases. Trips with David always had their zany side. We always almost missed the plane, the opening curtain and restaurant reservation. Still, I loved going places with David. Even when we were late, people rolled out the red carpet for my son.

For years, David and I had been talking about going to Europe together to visit Brussels, where I had grown up and spent World War II. I came of age speaking French; for many years my escape to fantasyland had consisted of burying myself in endless French novels. I knew and loved Paris long before I ever got there. A month before leaving for America, I had walked the familiar boulevards and bridges, rode the Metro, went to the Louvre, and necked with a French student in the Rodin museum. Each time I returned to Paris it felt as if I was coming home.

David and I finally went to Europe during the summer of 1990. He had preceded me, and welcomed me with a big bouquet of flowers at the Café des Deux Maggots, which adjoined our hotel. We shared our *café au lait* and croissants with Paris' sparrows.

I showed my son my favorite haunts: the Sainte Chapelle, Notre Dame, the Monuments des Deportés, the Louvre. I saw Paris with fresh eyes. I was making a superhuman effort to shelve my anxiety, but could not help worrying that David insisted on an afternoon nap. Fatigue was a symptom of full-blown AIDS. Years later, upon reading David's diaries, I discovered that after I retired for the night, he had gone out to dance half the night away. He went to a disco called "The Trap." The guys he met there, Luciano, Jacques, Patrick, were, as he wrote, "an embarrassment of riches." I smiled when I read the entries. It was as if David told me, "Mom, you see, while I was here I had a wonderful time."

After Paris we drove to Chartres, another one of my favorite places, then on to Bruges and Brussels. With David's customary thoroughness we located my school, and the many, many abodes where my family and I had lived and hid before, during and after World War II. One noon the Belgian family who had hidden me took us to an elegant lunch. Lucette, now nearing fifty, was born while I lived with her parents. I looked at her, her brother Jacques and their almost grown children and was happy and grateful.

Finally, the enchanted trip was over. I brought David to the airport, saw him mount a Sabena plane. Then I collapsed. How can one hurt so much, so soon after having been so happy? I sensed that a wondrous part of my life was gone forever.

5

AIDS IS CRAZY MAKING

Every Tuesday when I was in New York, I would journey to Greenwich Village and meet with my support group. Attendance now fluctuated between ten and fifteen, and sometimes we did not have enough chairs for everyone to sit on comfortably. We were like the AIDS quilt, so enormous by now that it took a fleet of trucks to cart it around America. Like the quilt panels, each mother was unique, yet the overall theme was remarkably uniform.

I had never been so intimately linked with so many women of such diverse backgrounds. We had all come to the group stunned by the unexpected misfortune that had descended on our families. We were angry, scared, bewildered, hopeful, surprised, guilty, incredulous and brave.

"Why me? Why him? Why us?" Sonia asked of no one in particular. Sonia's whole family had perished during the Holocaust. Now she was losing her only child to AIDS. "Did I not pay my dues? When is enough, enough?"

"I walked out on my husband and left my sons when they were in their teens," Inez told us. "Do you think that this is what made Eric gay? I wish that I could have AIDS instead of him," she sobbed. "Even so, I know that I could not have stayed with his father."

"If only that doctor had not insisted on that blood transfusion before he had surgery," Edith, a Long Island, accountant lamented.

"Adam said that he never had unprotected sex," Rhea said.

"I feel so stupid," Rona told the group. "I knew that Norm was gay, and I knew about AIDS, but I never put the two together." Rona, an elegant African-American woman, had flown in from Los Angeles as soon as she learned that her son was hospitalized with *pneumocystis pneumonia.*

"I do what Len asks me to do, even if I think it is silly," Laura reported in frustration. "And sometimes when it is done, he yells, and says that it is all wrong."

"If only I had not helped David fill out that application to Business School," I said.

Regret, self-incrimination, impotence, and introspection, however, only played a small part in our meetings. We were all there performing high-wire acrobatics. We helped our children live and die, hiding as best as we could our own grief, panic, and emotional fatigue. Most of us managed to seem optimistic and cheerful, even though our hearts were breaking. We all felt better when we vented our frustrations out loud and discovered that we were not unique.

Fran and Frank had retired, and Susan Katz, a veteran of the AIDS support community, now facilitated our meetings. Her involvement with AIDS had begun in 1981, when her 26-year old kid brother, Daniel, developed full-blown AIDS.

Susan had visited Daniel, the youngest of her three brothers, in California during the 1980s, about the time my David had moved there. The streets of San Francisco were filled with friendly people, gays, lesbians and flower children. People cross-dressed, danced and smoked marijuana. Sidewalk cafes overflowed with espresso, cappuccino, and Calistoga water. Daniel Katz was a friend of Armistead Maupin, whose *Tales of the City* mesmerized readers when they were printed in the *San Francisco Chronicle*. Mouse, one of the tale's most beloved characters, was modeled on Daniel Katz. No wonder that Susan, who lived in Kansas City, was captivated.

When Daniel became ill he moved back home to New York City to be near his parents. When Susan came to see him there, and realized how needy and weak he was, she stayed, helping her mother care for Dan during the last six months of his life. Daniel died in 1982, an early casualty of the disease.

For many of AIDS' "other" victims, the disease became a long-term commitment. Her hometown in Kansas and her thriving counseling practice no longer filled Susan's needs, and she too returned to New York to immerse herself in AIDS work. She became an AIDS counselor in an inner city clinic, created the first support group for mothers and sisters of HIV-positive hemophiliac patients, and trained AIDS workers at Hunter College. Earlier than most, Susan saw AIDS as a multi-generational epidemic, an infection that not only killed those it infected, but impacted the whole family, especially its women.

Like Fran Herman, Susan realized that women not only carried the physical brunt of caring for their sons, daughters, brothers, babies or husbands, but also suffered from emotional loss and guilt. This was sometimes coupled with abuse and financial hardship.

Susan, whose long red hair and petite figure made her look more like a college student than the 40-year old social worker she was, never did things half-heartedly. She devoted herself to the Mothers' Group, leading the Tuesday night meetings, providing individual counseling to some of the members and their children, making hospital visits and attending memorials. Once, when I commented on her dedication, she said:

"The group gives me more than I give it. It made me aware of the phenomenal resources of the women who belong to the group...I am in awe of what my own mother did for my brother...I pass on some of what I learn to the AIDS workers I train at Hunter..."

◆   ◆   ◆

In the beginning, the membership of the Mothers' Group consisted mostly of white, middle class women with gay sons. As the AIDS epidemic expanded, and disease increasingly spread to other risk groups, its social and ethnic make-up changed. One evening, in May 1988, Beverly Rotter arrived.

Tall, thin, blond and determined, Beverly Rotter described herself as a "single mother before this was commonplace." Beverly and her husband had split up when daughter Iris was seven and son Randy four. Social services and financial aid for single mothers were still in the future and Beverly made ends meet as best as she could.

She had taken any kind of job that came her way: hostessing, waitressing, transporting pets. "We lived in a family-oriented neighborhood and cared for each other's children," she recalled.

Beverly was proud of Iris, her daughter, who always had a project: writing, drawing, or caring for others. These were the 1960's, and Iris was a real flower child. At 17, long before she had developed any of her talents, she met and married Peter de la Cruz. By the time she was 18, Iris was a mother. At first Peter, Iris, and their daughter, Melissa, lived with Beverly, then they moved to Queens.

During the long, boring afternoons, Iris' neighbor turned her on to drugs. "I knew that Iris had an addictive personality," Beverly said. When Iris' habit escalated, Peter left. Iris and Melissa fended for themselves. Eventually Beverly took Melissa and sent Iris into a rehabilitation program.

Iris recovered and moved to Manhattan with Melissa. She still used drugs, but for many years was a functioning addict. Eventually, however, drugs landed Iris in jail. This time the rehabilitation worked, and after her tumultuous life as a single mother, prostitute, writer, and drug-user, 36-year-old Iris found respectable employment as an emergency medical technician. Beverly started relaxing about her daughter.

Iris worked for the medical emergency service and criss-crossed Manhattan aboard an ambulance. She loved her job and ignored her tiredness and even the "white stuff" that occasionally filled her mouth. Iris could not, however, ignore a persistent high fever. When it spiked at 105.5°, she went to the emergency room and was hospitalized. Three months later, Iris knew she had AIDS. She was very thin and looked, as she wrote in her memoirs, "like the national AIDS poster child." She moved back home to Brooklyn, "feeling unloved and unclean," and prepared to die.

Beverly would not let Iris die. She collected and read all the information pertaining to AIDS that she could find, including an issue of the PWAC (People With Aids Coalition) Newsline, which listed the mothers' support group.

Beverly' came to the meeting, but decided not to come back. "Who needs to listen to everyone else's horror stories and troubles," she told her daughter when she got home. Iris, who by then had intermittent seizures, felt that her mother would not make it on her own. She insisted that Beverly return to the group the following Tuesday. Very quickly Beverly responded to the group's healing power.

"It was the one place where I could let it all out," Beverly recalled. "I knew nobody else infected by the HIV virus. I had nobody to talk to about AIDS. I worked in a restaurant, and was afraid that if they found out about Iris, they would fire me."

At the group Beverly was given a list of doctors treating AIDS. She and Iris selected Dr. Jeffrey Greene, one of New York's most beloved AIDS specialists. Greene put Iris on AZT and prescribed antibiotics and vitamins. Under Greene's care, Iris improved. Her seizures stopped, she gained weight, looked beautiful, and now put all her energies into fighting AIDS. "She worked twenty out of twenty-four hours," her mother remembers.

Both Beverly and Iris had leadership qualities. Beverly assumed an important role in the Mothers' Group, organizing many of its off-site activities. She was a professional Jewish mother and comforted us with food. More importantly, she knew how to talk tough, and taught other members to be assertive with doctors, nurses and other health care workers.

After a period of locking herself up at home, Iris started attending a group for HIV-positive women, also meeting in "The Living Room" of the house in Greenwich Village. When the facilitator of that group became too ill to continue, Iris took over.

During the 1970's, while she was hustling on Third Avenue, Iris wrote columns on drugs and sex for men's magazines. Now she used her pen and energy battling AIDS: writing about safer sex, urging addicts to clean up their act, and living a day at a time. She also started writing her autobiography. In 1990, men still accounted for the majority of the "visible" AIDS patients. But, as Iris realized:

> "…there were other women with the virus. There were black women and white women, Latinas, rich women and poor women. There were addicts and transfusion women. They were mothers, sisters and lovers and grandmothers…Outside differences became trivial; survival was every one's main concern."

(from *Women, AIDS & Activism,* South End Press, 1990.)

Iris also discovered love in her own heart. She renewed her bonds with her mother and nineteen-year-old Melissa. Iris made new friends and even planned to marry another PWA (person with AIDS.) She set a May date for the wedding and picked a sexy wedding dress. When the group heard about Iris' wedding plans, it shook its collective head in disbelief. We knew that Iris' health was declining, and we feared that by May she would really be ill.

When I saw Iris in December 1990, AIDS had suddenly transformed this vibrant woman into a tortured creature waiting at death's door. A few months earlier she had developed early signs of dementia, and within weeks AIDS took over her entire body. In January she tried to escape from Beverly's loving confine. One day when she felt very ill, she left Brooklyn on her own and went to the emergency room at New York University Medical Center. Iris, who had taught dozens of People with AIDS how to navigate successfully the red tape, sat there helplessly until Beverly came to the rescue. Within days after this expedition Iris was hospitalized and slipped into a coma. Beverly had promised her that she would be in "no pain" at the end. The physician ordered a morphine drip. The end was near. Mothers trooped to the hospital for support.

As evening approached, the staff wanted to get rid of the three mothers who had stayed with Beverly. Deane successfully dug in her heels, declaring that they were not going to let that "mother face her daughter's death alone."

A few weeks later we all gathered to bid Iris farewell. The small chapel was filled with Iris' family, friends and many of those whom she had touched during her stormy life. The Union of the Prostitutes of New York (P.O.N.Y.) established a scholarship in her memory and New York City named its new home and treatment center for women with AIDS Iris House.

Iris' death in 1991—four months before her hoped-for wedding—marked a major change in the Mothers' Group. Until then all the mothers met in the "downstairs" Living Room. Now Beverly insisted that mothers whose children had died would meet in the "upstairs" room of the little house. "We no longer have the same problems," Beverly said. "We have lost the battle, and are jealous of those of you who still have hope." The stairs that separated "upstairs" from "downstairs" became a vivid symbol of the finality AIDS.

◆   ◆   ◆

Rhea Parham joined the group a year before Iris' death. She arrived one Tuesday in February, because Adam, her only child, was infected with the HIV virus. At first she was totally distraught by what she witnessed, but the strength of the group buoyed her up.

Everybody's reaction to tragedy is different. Some people become totally absorbed by their personal misery. Others become nasty and abusive. Rhea managed to grow with her pain, and even had strength left for others. No matter how depressed she was, her open smile was like a ray of sun on a gray day.

It was impossible to believe that at his birth Rhea had almost given Adam up for adoption. When Rhea was 19, she had left her loving, somewhat overprotective, parents in Brooklyn and moved to Los Angeles. There she fell in love with Enrico, an aspiring actor and cab driver. He was rather volatile. Within months Rhea and Enrico had a terrible fight. After Rhea had returned to New York she discovered that she was pregnant.

She called Enrico, and they decided to get married. All seemed well. Rhea told her parents, bought a wedding dress and arranged a small party. The wedding was not to be. Enrico called and told Rhea that he just could not go through with it.

In 1966, nice middle-class Jewish girls did not have children out of wedlock. Rhea's parents declined to help. Rhea felt that she could not manage on her own. There was a great demand for Jewish babies, and Rhea contacted the Louise Wise Adoption Service. No doubt this reputable agency would find a highly qualified childless couple that would provide her baby with a better chance in life than she herself could. Rhea moved to a home for unwed mothers on Staten Island, and her baby was born at a nearby hospital. Rhea recalled:

"I gave birth on a Friday. My father came to see my baby boy and me in the hospital, crying about the two of us. I knew Dad had always wanted a son."

Rhea had signed preliminary adoption papers. The agency had told her that they had placed her son with a suitable family on Long Island.

"On Monday I moved back to my parents' house, bidding my child farewell." Rhea continued. "A week later I returned to the hospital to visit a friend who had just given birth. To my utter surprise my son was still there, stuck in his hospital crib. I felt that the agency had lied to me about the placement."

Terribly angry, Rhea picked up her baby and returned to her parents' house.

"They had a change of heart and told me they would help. My mother could not look at Adam for six months, but my father and my grandmother surrounded him with love. Adam and my father grew wonderfully close. Even after Dad died, Adam said that he could still smell him and feel his beard against his chin."

Realizing that one could still be with a person even if he or she had died turned out to be a great consolation for both Rhea and Adam.

Years later, when Rhea told Adam about the near-adoption, he had said, "Mom, I could not have lived if I had not known you. I would not have fitted."

Rhea and Adam grew up together. "From early on, Adam was both cautious and independent." Rhea recalled. "Once he had investigated something and decided he wanted it, he went after it full blast. I never treated him like a baby. He understood that I had to get on with my life. I needed him to be self-reliant, and he was.

Adam was always in a hurry, as if he knew he did not have much time. He loved good things—food, clothes, going places—and worked so he could afford them. At 11, he bussed in a restaurant. At 12 he knew that he wanted to be an actor. He enrolled at the Henry Street Settlement House, joined a stage crew and sold theater programs.

He attended New York's High School for the Performing Arts, becoming romantically involved with both boys and girls, always wondering whether he was gay or straight.

Adam modeled and landed small roles in television soaps. In 1982, when he was 19, Adam moved to Los Angeles and tried to break into the movies, capturing an occasional assignment, supporting himself as before by working in restaurants. He had arrived in California in the midst of a hepatitis epidemic, and got himself vaccinated.

In 1987 Adam realized that his medical insurance had lapsed. When he applied for a new policy, the company required an HIV test. It was positive! The people at the testing center told him that he would be dead in six months! Since Adam had always practiced "safe sex" he believed that his infection stemmed from the hepatitis vaccination.

Before telling his Mom and his friends about his illness, Adam tried to come to terms with the deadly disease. He went to San Cristobal in Mexico, a very spiritual place, practiced Aikido and meditated. Thanksgiving, 1989, he came to New York and told Rhea about being HIV-positive.

"I freaked out," Rhea recalled. "I had already lost three friends to AIDS. I thought I would lose him anytime. I was frightened and scared.

"Adam managed to reassure me. He gave me Bernie Segal's book *Love, Medicine and Miracles* to read, and told me that he was not going to die then and there. He taught me to take it one day at a time." Then Adam returned to California.

The next summer Rhea went out to Los Angeles to help Adam move to a new apartment. When she saw her son, she knew that he was quite ill. He was skinny, ran a fever of 105°, had thrush, and his T-cells were dropping. His throat was eroded by an ulcer, which his doctor was treating with borax, peroxide and vitamin C infusions.

"'Adam, are you going to handle this illness all by yourself?'" Rhea asked him. "'Come home to Brooklyn.'"

"Adam must have been very vulnerable," Rhea reflected, "because he agreed. We packed in a hurry, shipped 26 cartons by railway express, sold his car, and were on our way."

In New York, Adam consulted Dr. Greene, who had done so much for Iris. Whether it was love or better medical care, within weeks after his arrived in New York Adam got better and regained his weight. Even his throat ulcer yielded to an antifungal cream.

The AIDS virus did not let Adam relax for long. Within a few months he again developed a high fever, headaches, nausea and vomiting. Rhea accompanied him to the emergency room at Long Island Hospital.

Adam suffered from *cryptococcal meningitis* (CM), a condition in which the *cryptococcus* fungus inflamed the membrane that covers the brain and the spinal cord. Like most opportunistic infections, CM was rare in the pre-AIDS days. After a critical few weeks, Adam recovered.

Dr. Leonard Berkowitz, an infectious disease specialist, and now another one of New York's over-busy AIDS physicians, had treated Adam in the hospital and continued to care for him. Dr. Berkowitz was impressed by Adam's courage—his determination to live a full life in spite of AIDS.

Some AIDS patients go to the doctor only when absolutely necessary. Others, like Adam, and my son David, explored every possibility. Both Rhea and Adam read constantly about AIDS, subscribing to numerous newsletters. Adam was very much his own physician. Berkowitz respected his determination, and sometimes simply acted as if he were Adam's consultant.

Like David Loebl, Adam tried every available cure: Egg lipids, Chinese herbs, dextran sulfate, and St. John's wort, also know as Compound Q. In 1991, the highly toxic herb, extracted from a Chinese cucumber, was touted to be a possible AIDS cure. In spite of its ambiguous legal status, Compound Q was available at some buyers' clubs. Adam located his weed in Texas.

When injected, Compound Q can cause high fever, chills, anaphylactic shock, or respiratory failure. Rhea watched as a reluctant Berkowitz injected the preparation. After each treatment, Rhea and Adam left the doctor's office with three filled syringes: one full of cortisone to counteract anaphylactic shock, one with epinephrine to overcome respiratory failure, and one full of decadron, meant to alleviate mental confusion. These emergency measures were unnecessary, but the drug caused high fevers, chills and such severe muscle pain that Adam could not get out of bed for a day or two after the injection. After several months he gave up.

People struggling with AIDS want time to stand still. Like me, many mothers found a special closeness with their infected children and treasured every shared moment. Unfortunately, these intense interactions stress other meaningful relationships. Rhea's long-standing relationship with Donald L. disintegrated, partly because she put all her energies into helping her son. Rhea also lost the house into which she had sunk her life's savings. She had to look for new quarters for herself and Adam.

Rhea rented a small apartment in Brooklyn. Adam obtained a studio in the Manhattan Center in Manhattan, a low-rent housing complex, in which some apartments were earmarked for AIDS patients. Broadway Cares, the AIDS arm of Actor's Equity, not only paid the rent but also provided him with excellent health insurance.

Rhea and Adam were overjoyed. Adam was happy to have his own space, and Rhea too welcomed the distance. Rhea threw Adam a big house-warming party. His well-equipped household was a testimonial to the generosity of his and Rhea's many friends.

Because of his own positive outlook, Adam managed to emotionally sustain other AIDS patients. He made new friends, including Pam Shaw, the shy, HIV-positive stepdaughter of Carol, a faithful group member. Her first lover had infected Pam heterosexually. She was healthy, even though she only had seven T-cells.

Before she met Adam, Pam was utterly depressed and carefully hid her HIV status. Adam opened Pam's closet. The beautiful, blue-eyed, blond woman now looked the world straight in the face, stating by her mere appearance that "If I, a heterosexual, white college student can contract AIDS, so can your sons and daughters." Soon Pam Shaw became a darling of the television talk shows, and a feature in popular glossy magazines. AIDS would kill her, but she made a difference in the world's fight against this disease.

◆   ◆   ◆

Lynn joined the Mothers' Group in 1991. Her 28-year-old son, Paul—a drug user—had tested positive for HIV. Lynn was a petite, sweet and innocent-looking woman. One wonders how she coped with the crass drug world. During her first evening at the group she told us her story:

"We lived in a middle-class neighborhood in Queens. When Paul was a junior in high school I noticed that he sometimes was not quite there. His father was drinking, so I assumed that Paul was a chip off the old block and was also drinking. 'Thank God,' I told myself, 'it isn't drugs.'" But Paul was not drinking. He was mainlining heroin. He was 17 years old.

"When I found out that it was drugs," Lynn said, "I felt as if somebody had stuck a knife into me. When I recovered from the initial shock, I thought, like every drug-user's mother, that I could make my kid quit. But you can't make them stop. Eventually you realize that they'll quit only when they want to.

"I made Paul get into detox. It did work for a while, but he always went back onto drugs. He supported his habit by breaking into cars. Once I forbade him to come home and he was arrested. He was sent to Riker's Island (New York City's Municipal prison) where he learned the tricks of the trade.

"Paul was arrested and sent to Riker's three times in a row. When he was released he was drug-free for a while, then start drugging again. By 1986 all inmates were tested for the AIDS virus, and in 1986 and in 1987 Paul was HIV-negative. We talked about AIDS, and he assured me that he was using new needles.

"He did not stick to his promise. Sometimes in 1991 he must have gotten so desperate for a fix that he shared (needles). He got very sick; developed blood poisoning and endocarditis (inflammation of the membrane surrounding the heart.) He was hospitalized and tested positive for HIV.

"It has been rough since. Initially he refused to keep his doctor's appointments. He hated being sick. He said, 'Look at Rock Hudson and Liberace. They had all the money in the world and got the best care. They still died, so what is the difference?'

"Now, I think that we've turned a corner," Lynn continued. "Paul has stuck with his methadone program. He went from a maintenance dose of 80 mg/day down to 10mg/day. In a couple of months he'll be completely off.

"We finally found a woman doctor Paul likes, and he is clean, I believe for good. Now he is taking responsibility for his own health. He keeps track of his T-cell count and was proud when it went up from 240 to 360. He said the other day: 'I thought I had problems before. Now I know what a real problem is.'

"I am grateful." Lynn told us. "I have a wonderful new, supportive husband, and I have Vinnie, my warm, gentle gay son. He is my best friend and he promised that he would help me take care of his brother."

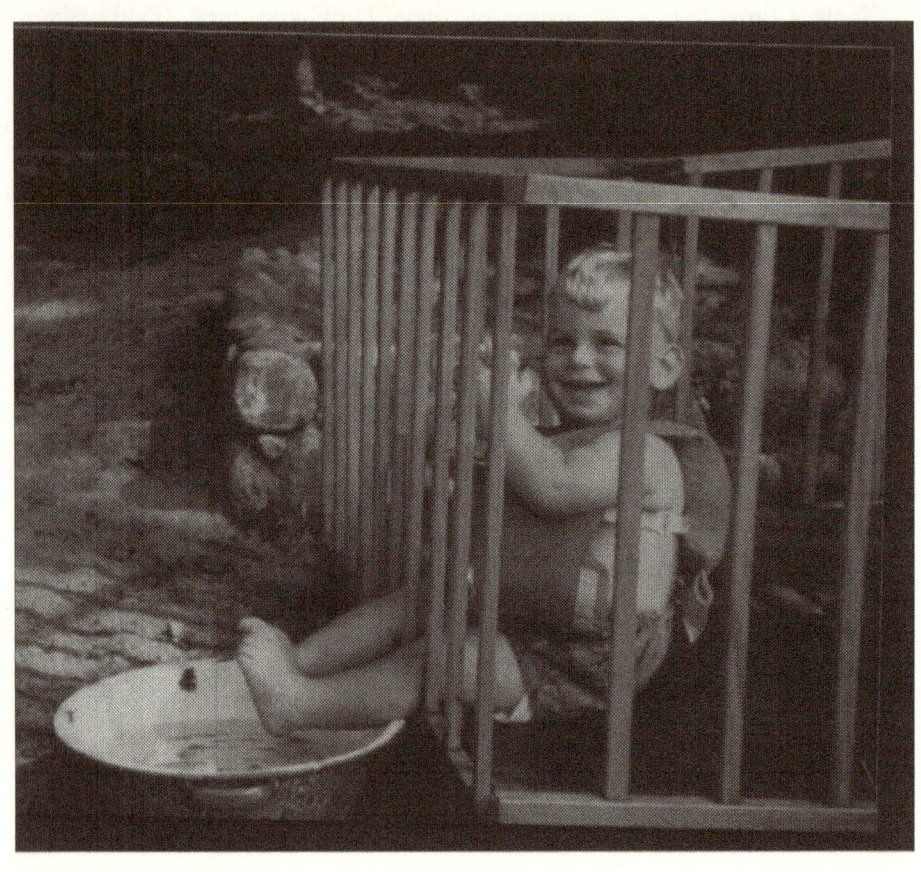

David in 1957

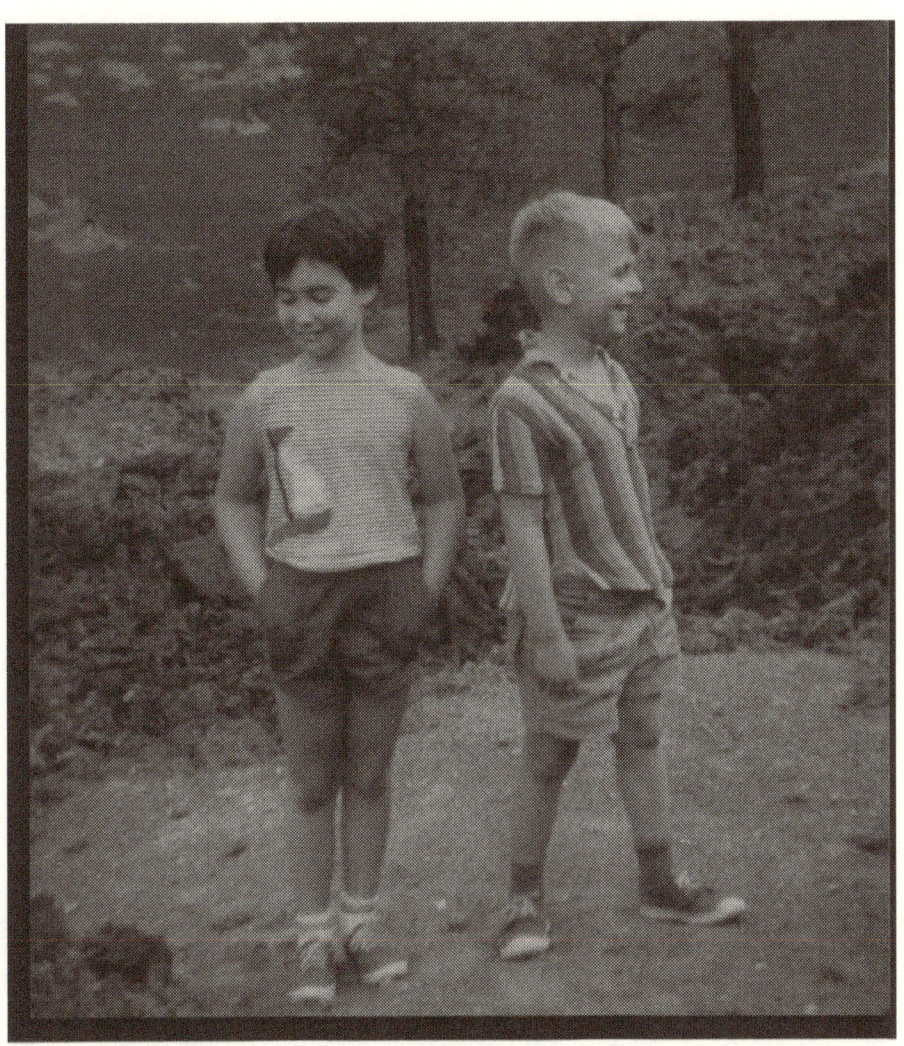

Judy and David Loebl

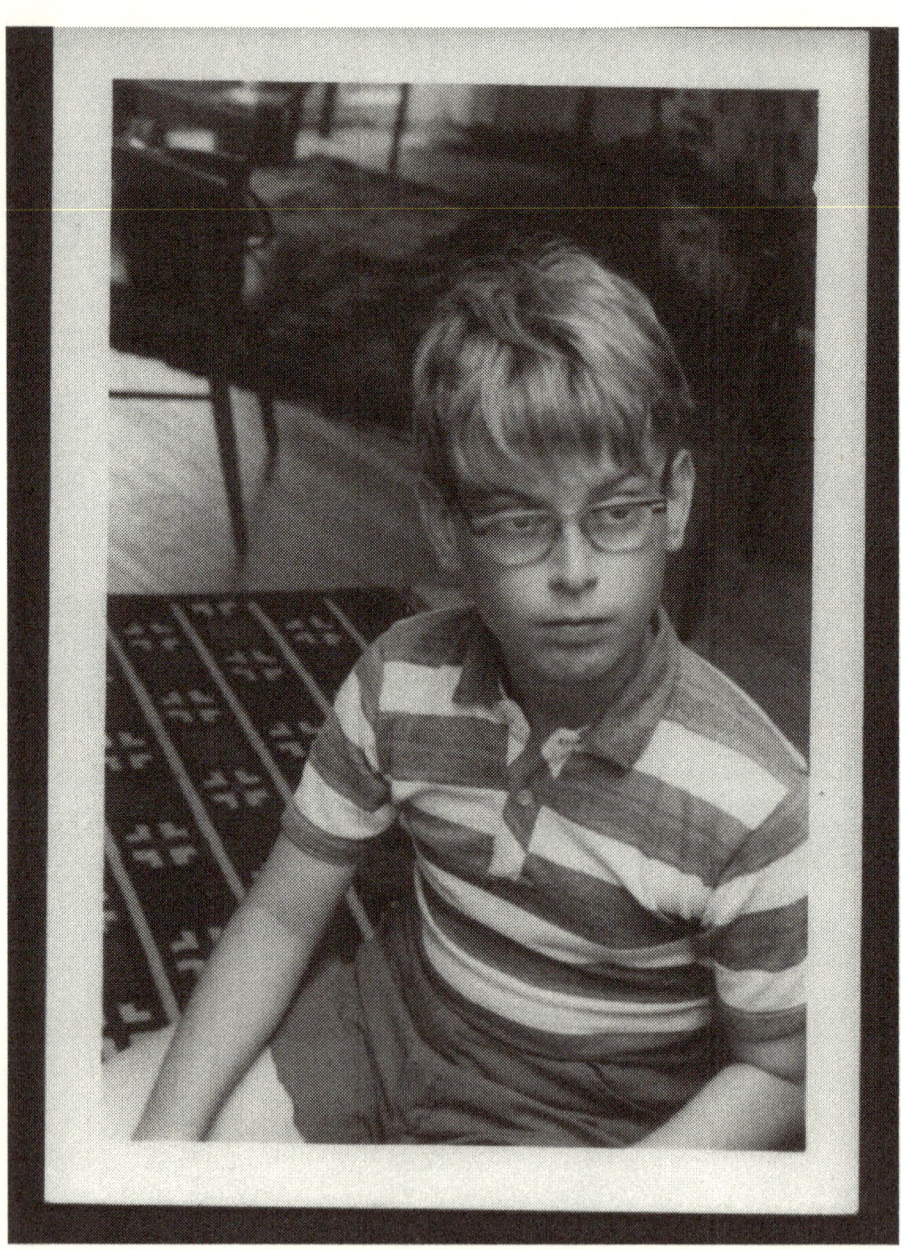

David

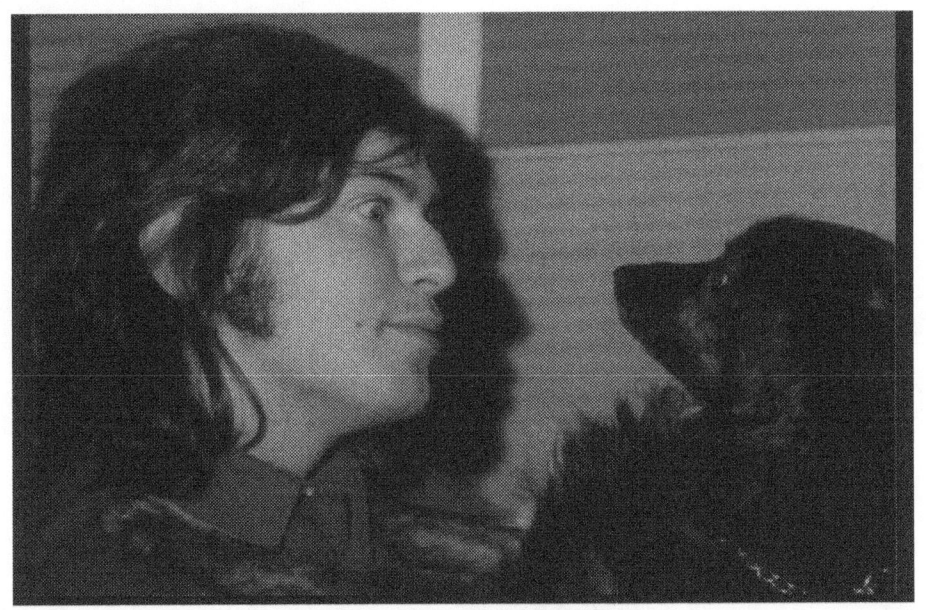

David and Shirley at Brandeis

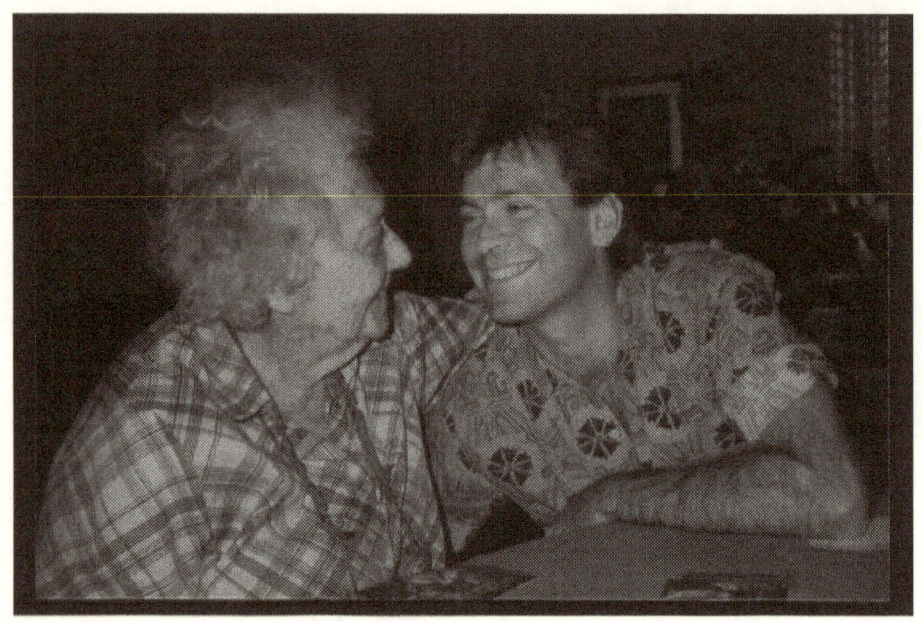

David and his beloved grandmother

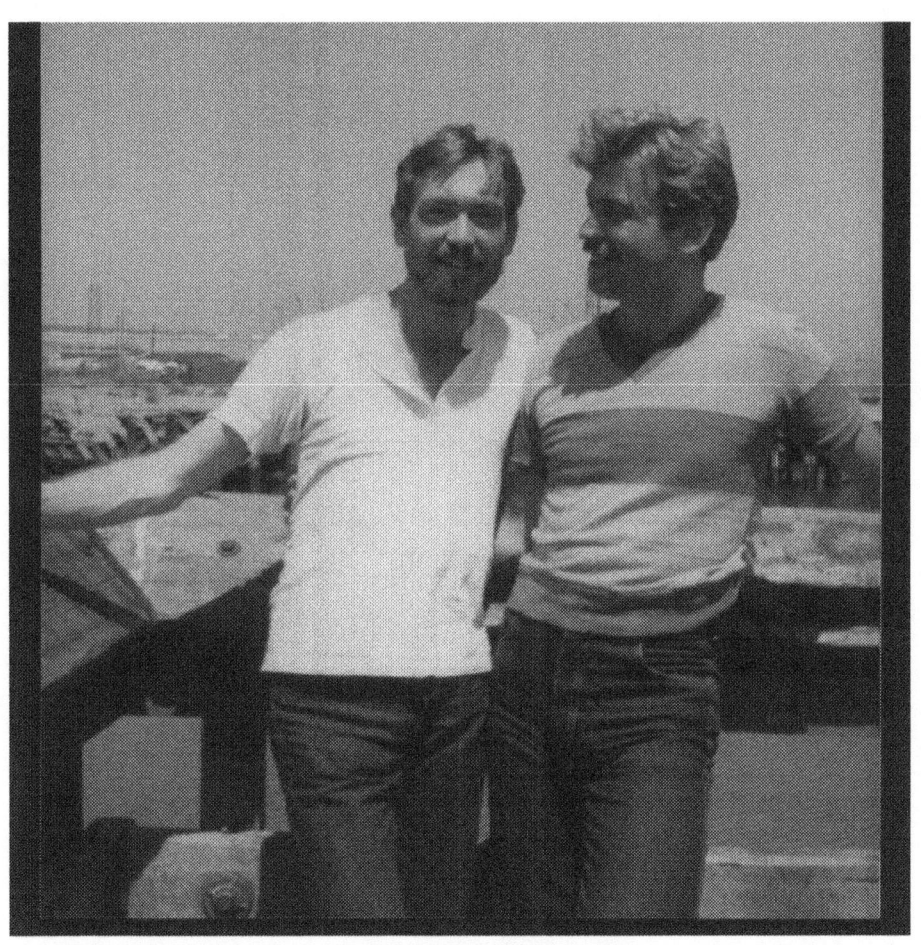

Joseph Ahern and David

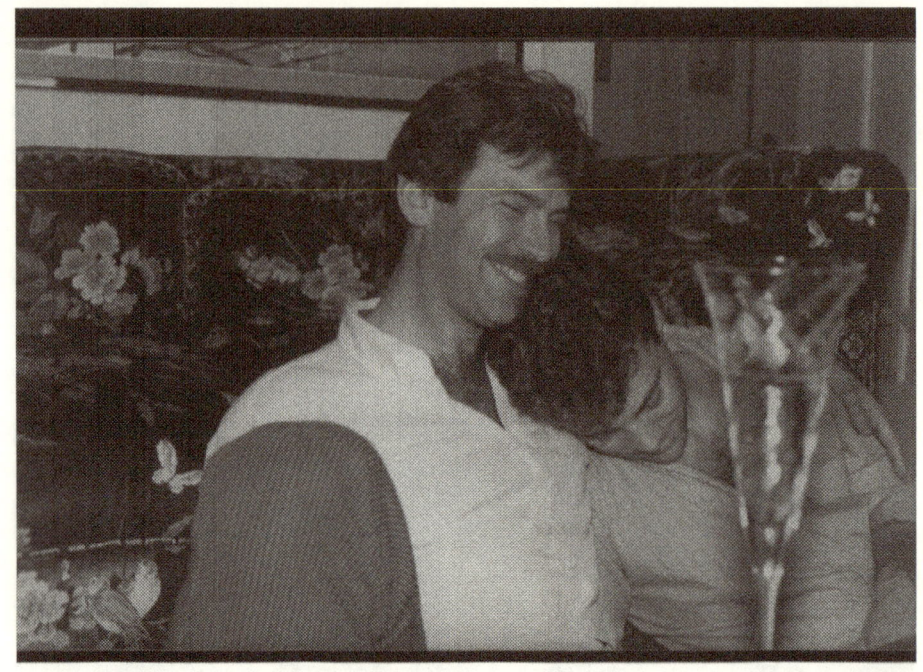

David and Jeff Price

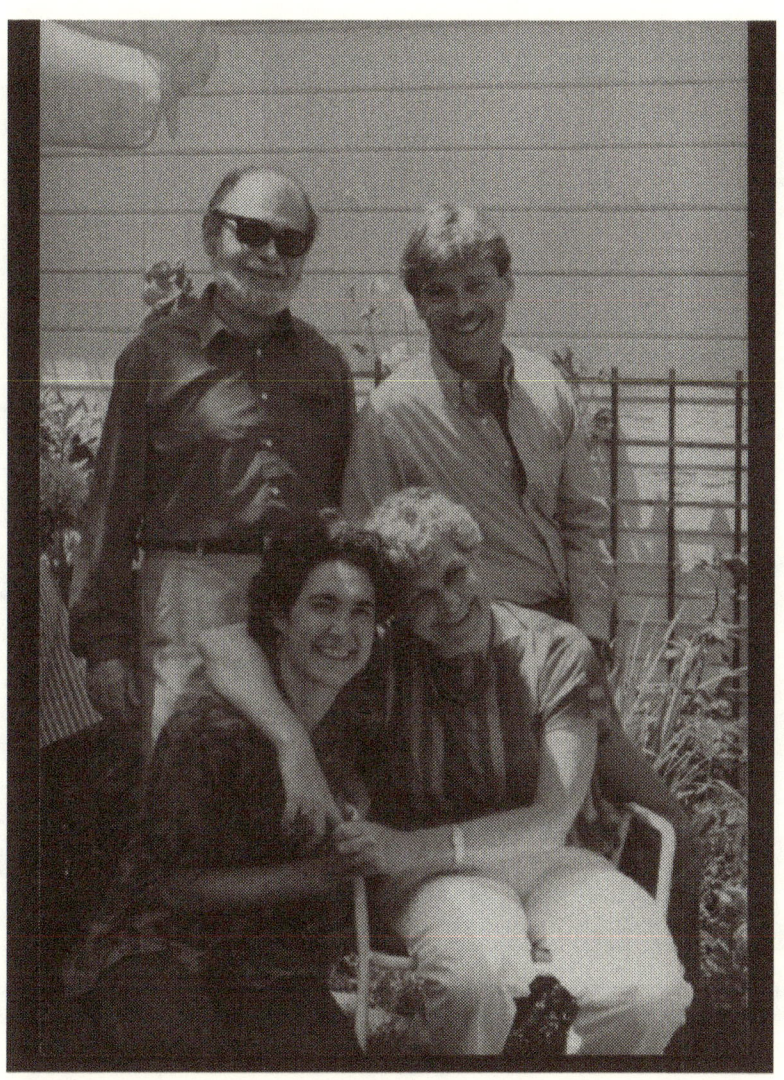

The four Loebls at David's graduation

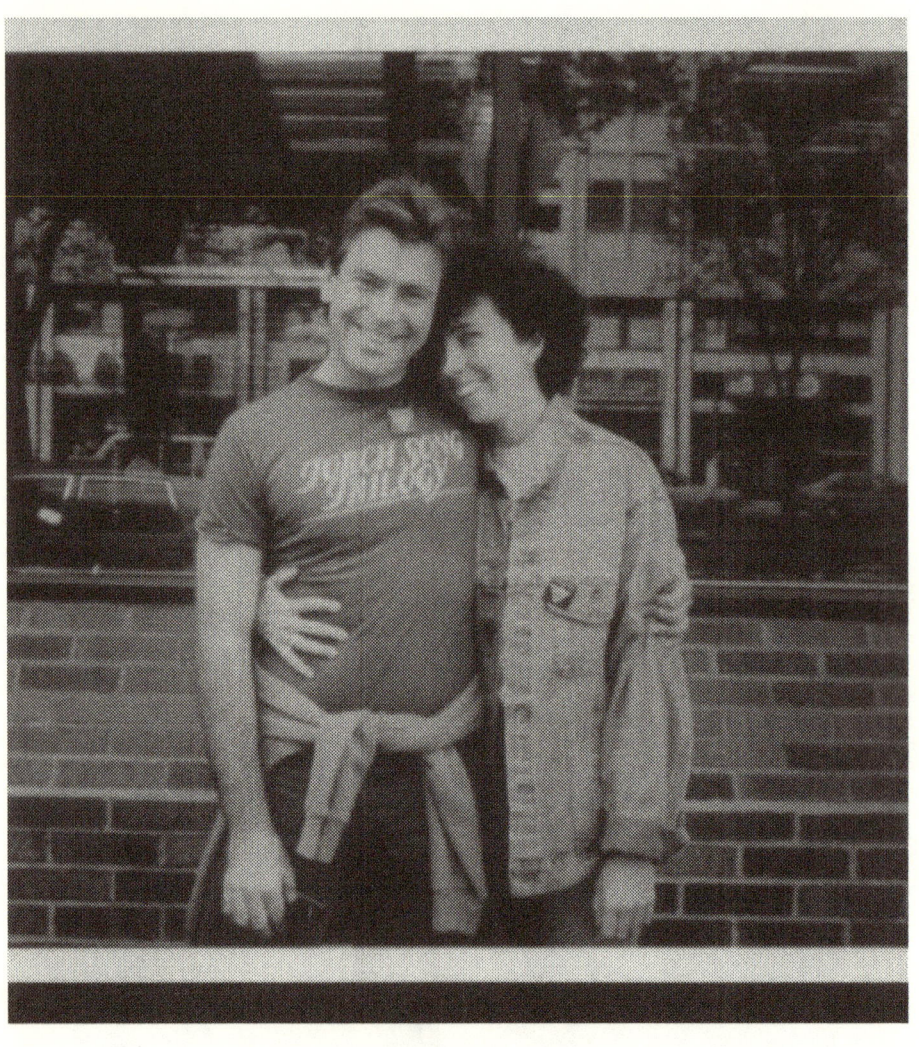

David and Andrea Lepcio

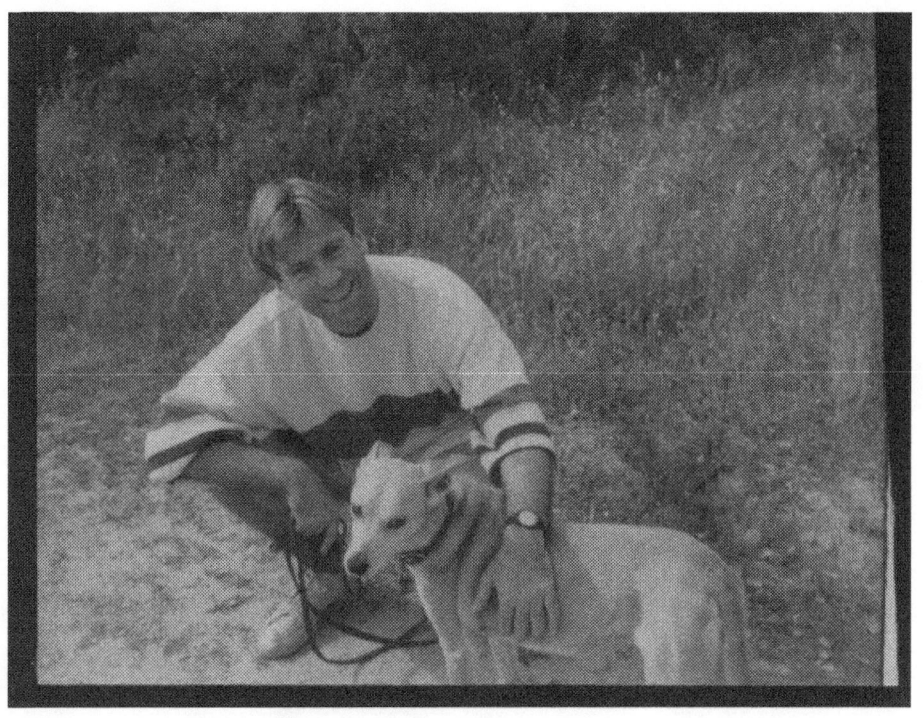

David and Liza

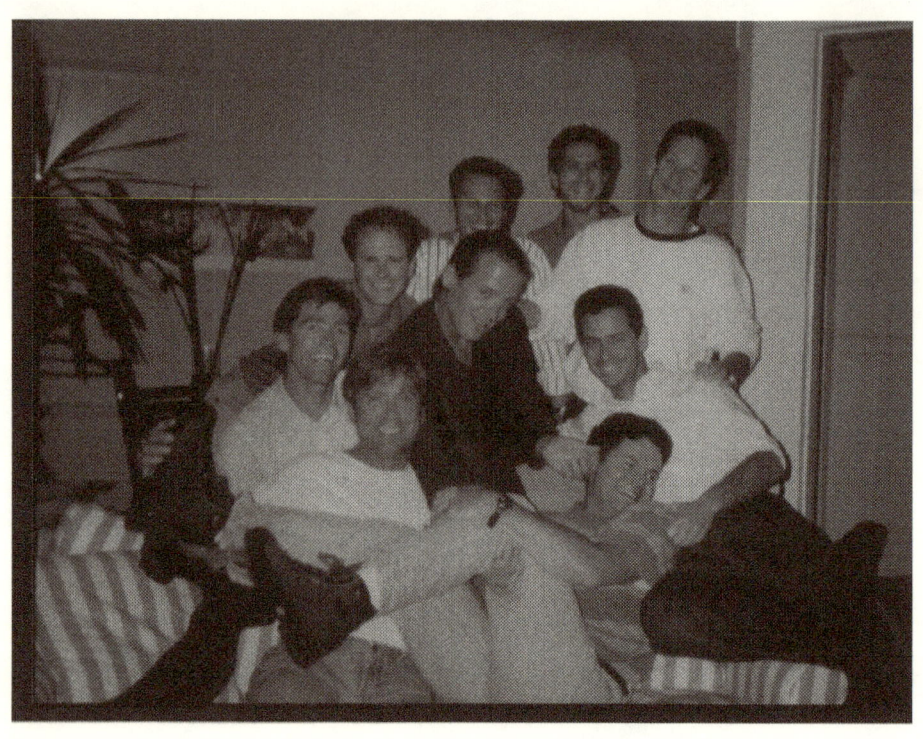

David and his gang in San Francisco

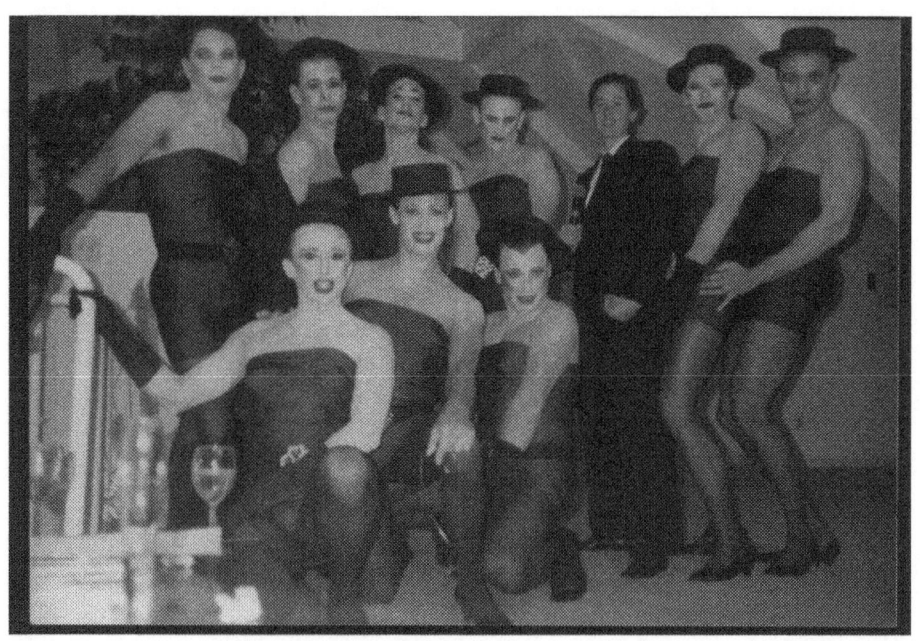

David at Halloween

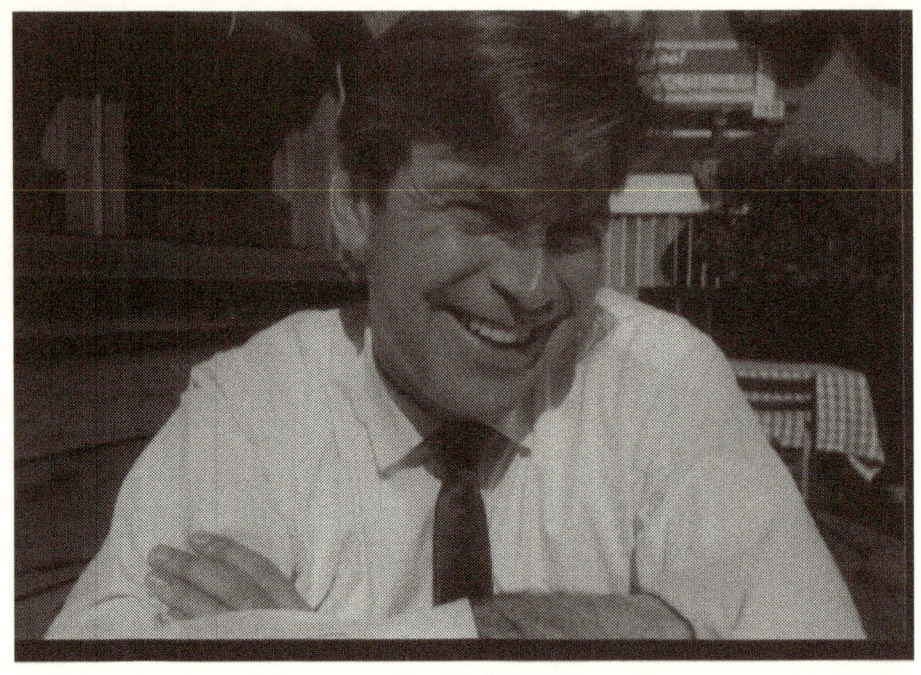

Lunch at Baywulf in Oakland

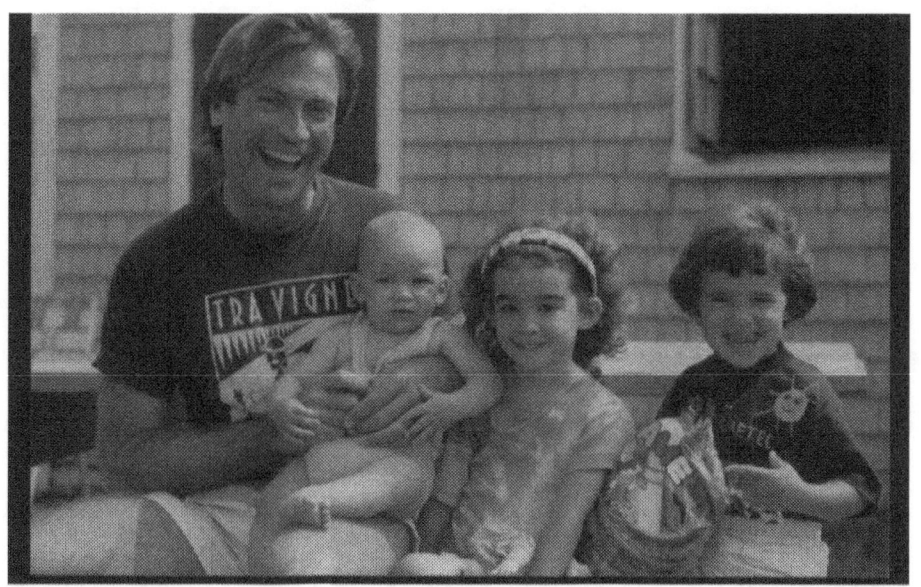

With Sean, Ana and Naomi

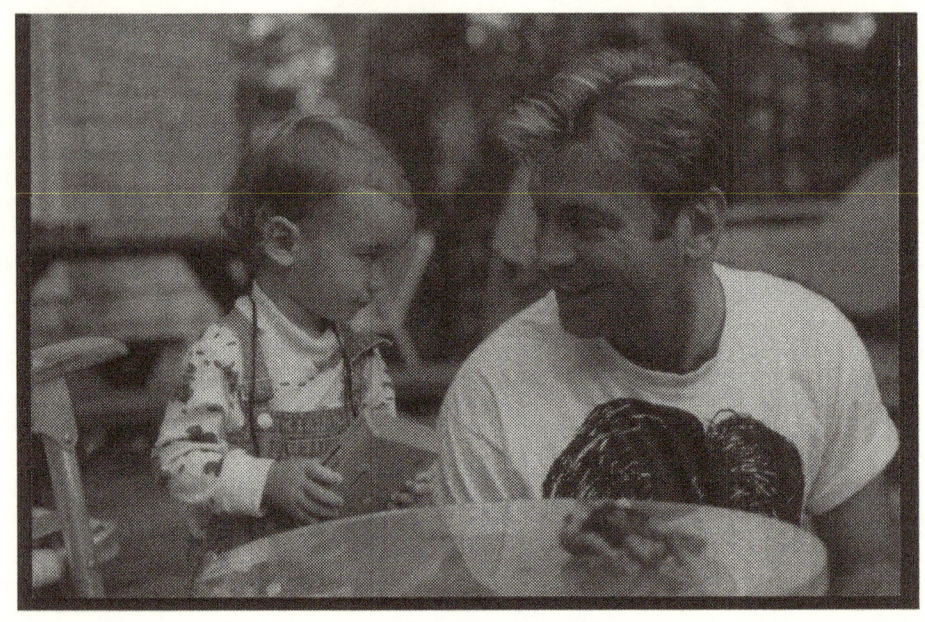

David and Sean

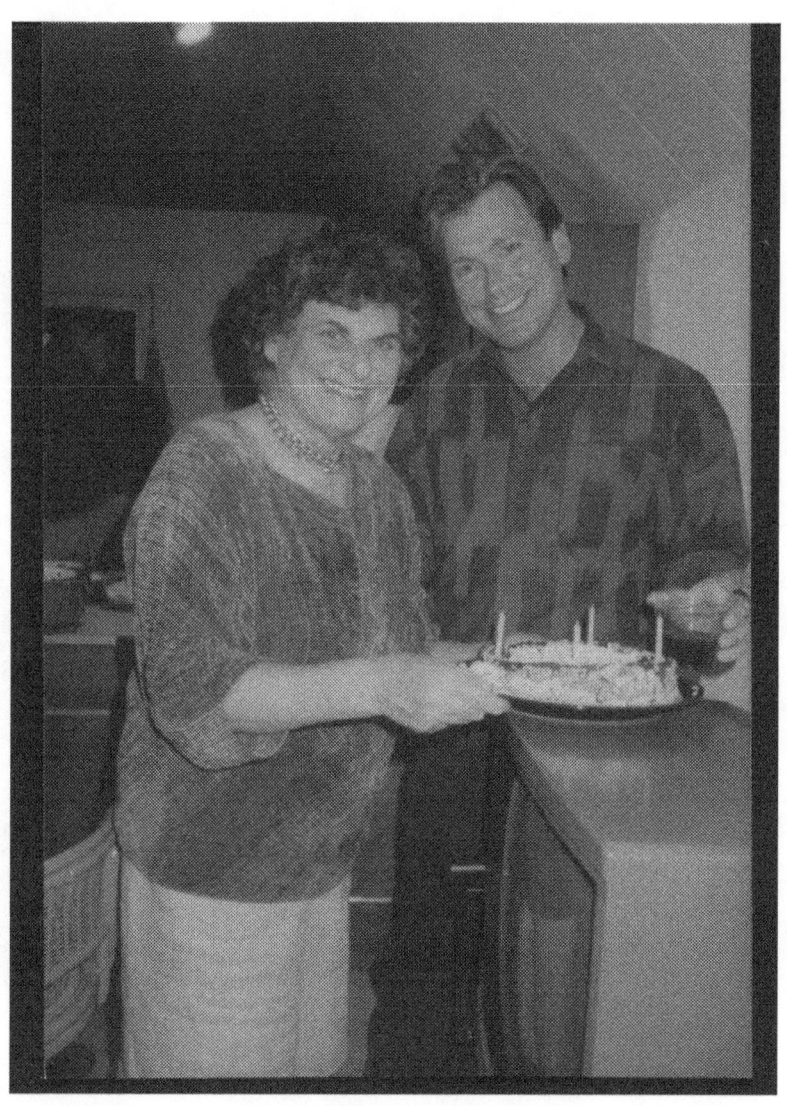

Suzanne and David at his 37th birthday

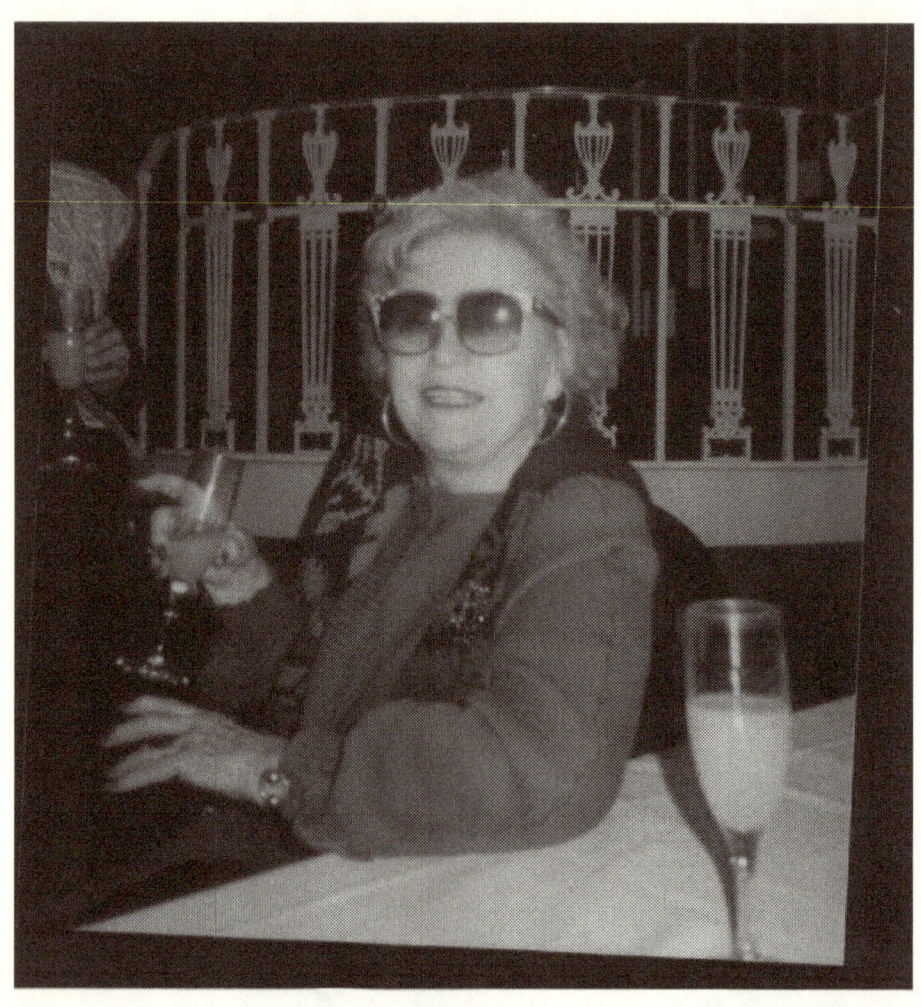

Deane Dixon

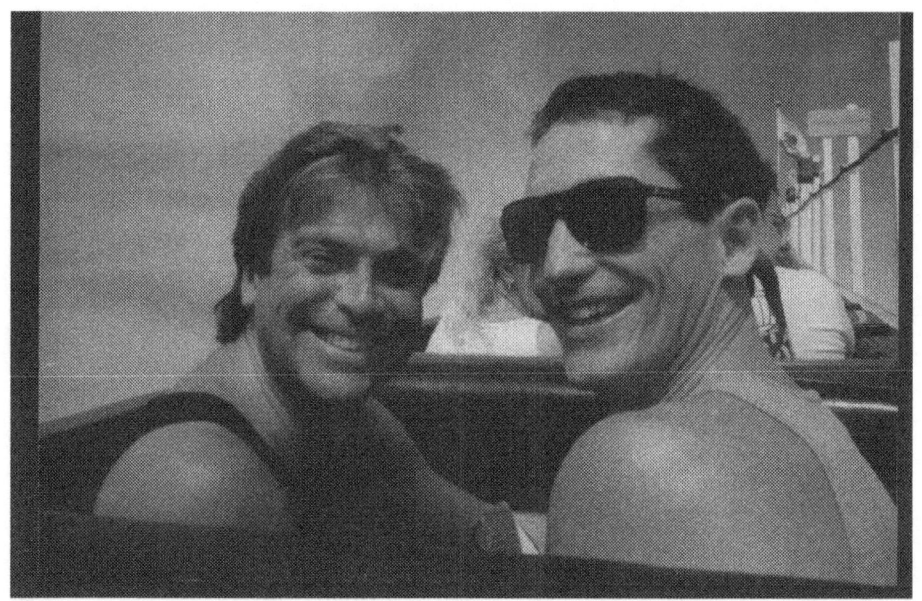

David and his friend Frank

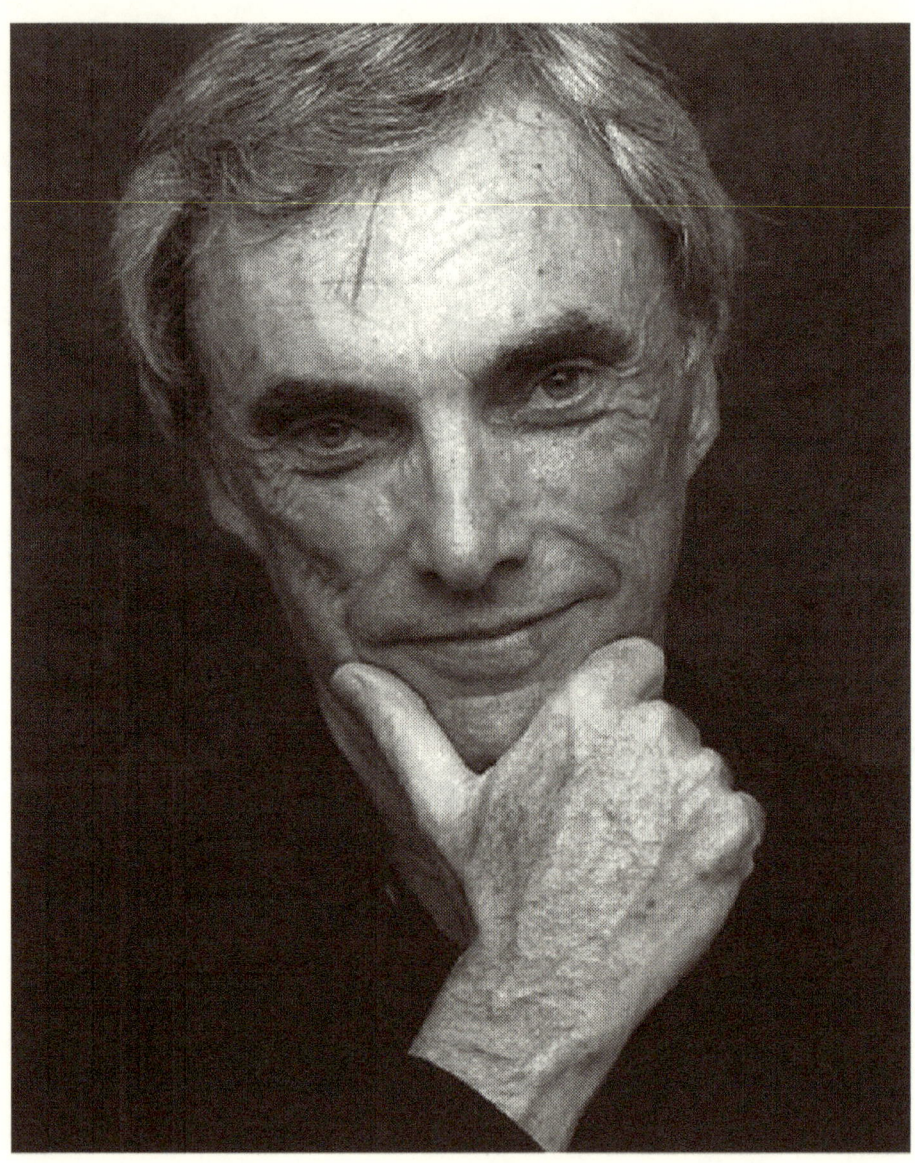

Frank Donnelly

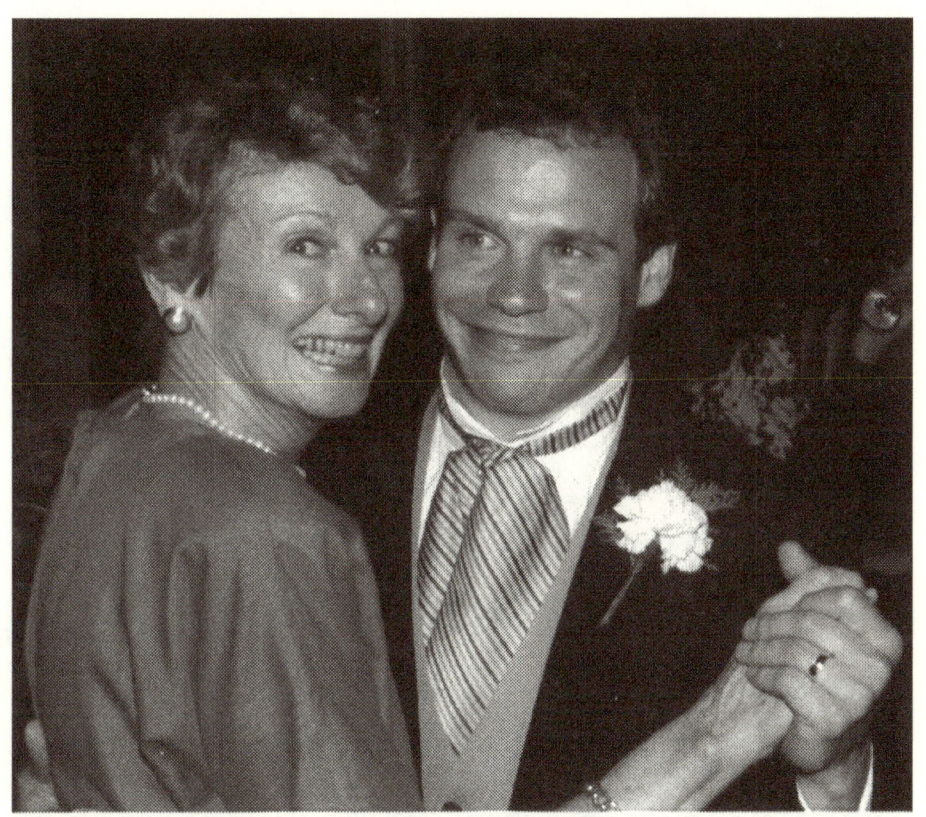

Maggie and Patrick J.

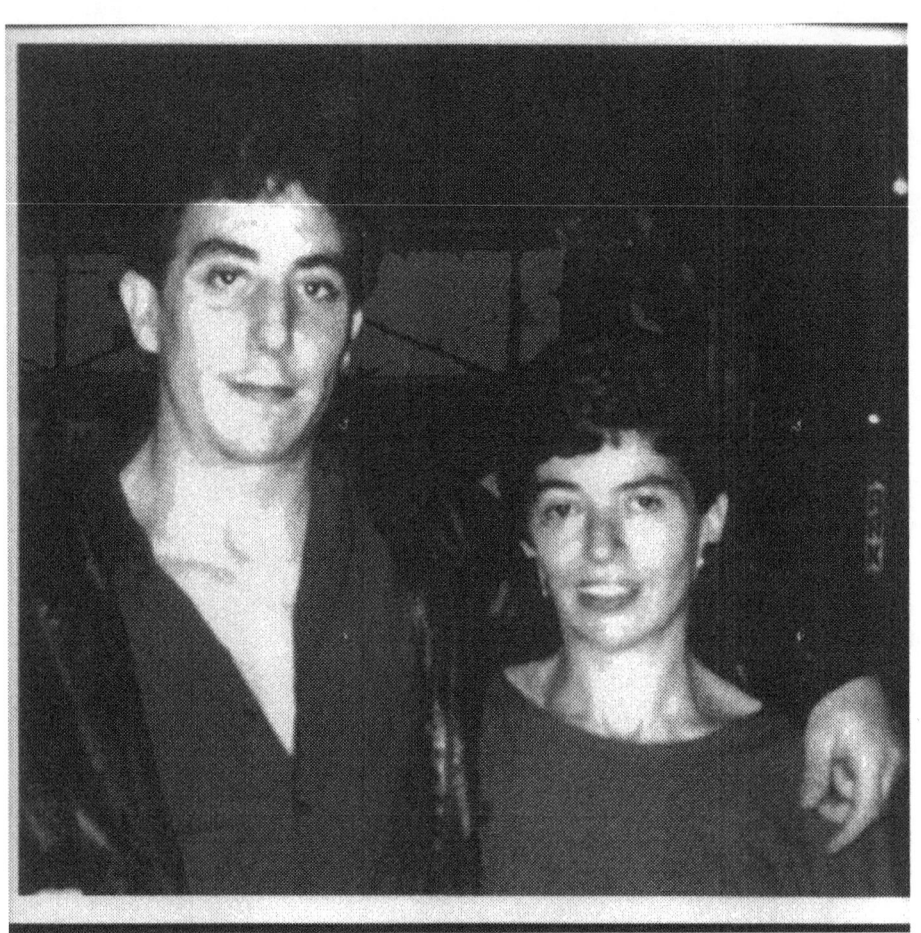

Brian Misciagna and Blanche Mednick

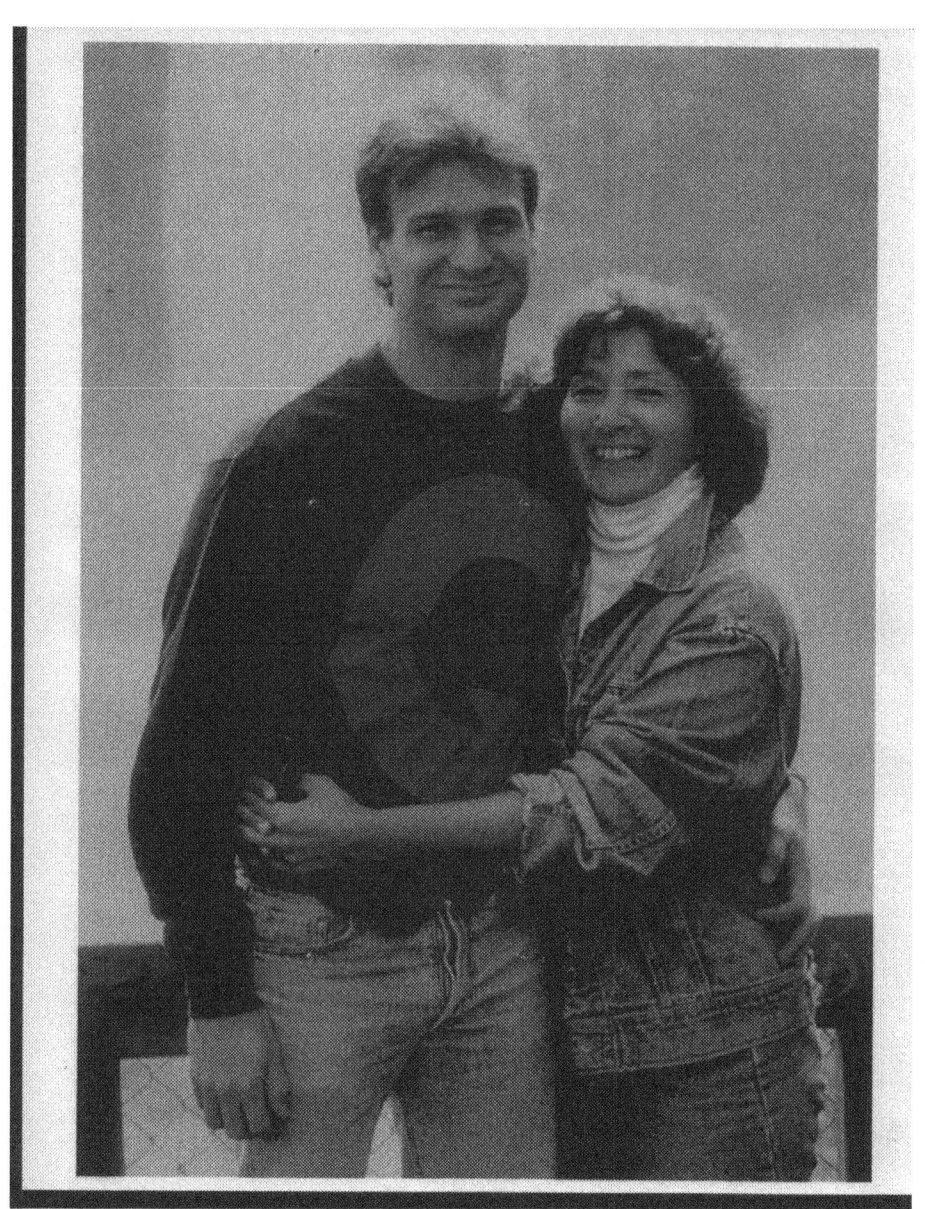

Adam Balzano and Rhea Cohen

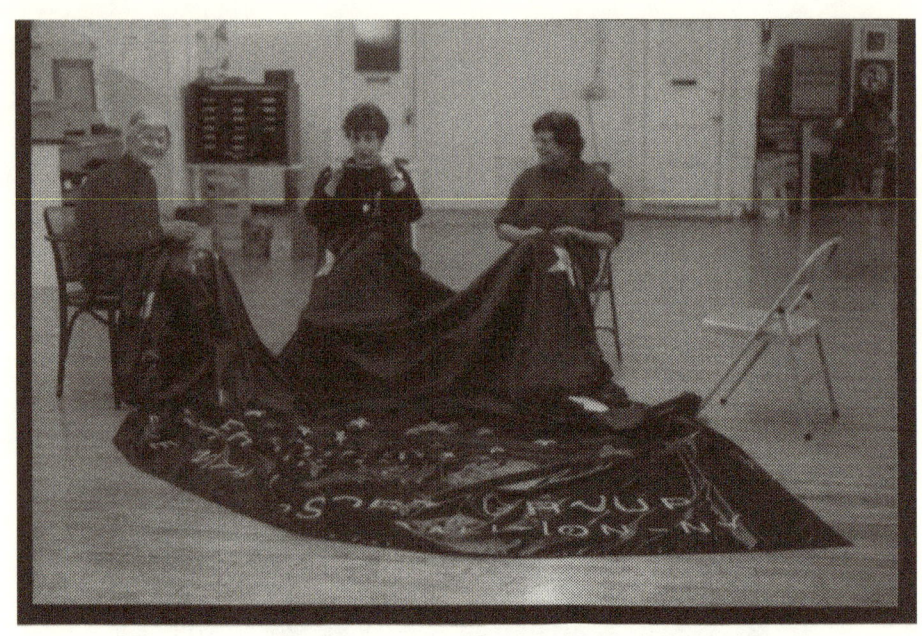

Sewing stars on the Mothers' Group Quilt

6

TO WISH UPON A STAR

I had barely arrived in California in February 1991, when, two weeks before her 89th birthday, my mother died. When I told David he screamed. We were to fly to New York, for my Mom's funeral, but first David went off to his office, to finish some pressing work. He was sobbing.

"It feels good to cry, for once, about something so acceptable as the death of a grandmother," he told me after he got home.

More people came to my mom's funeral than I had expected. To my extended family, my mother had been a last link to what Jewish life had been in Germany before the Holocaust. My cousins always had admired my mother's charisma and her free spirit. But then they never had to deal with her mercurial changes of mood, her self-involvement, her pride and her stubbornness.

My relationship with my mother had been complex and intense. She blew hot and cold. One day she was loving and seductive; then, without warning, she was rejecting and dissatisfied. She was a loner, but demanded my devotion. She was domineering and vulnerable. She was needy and proud. I was her emotional support for as long as I can remember, even though we both resented this close entanglement. During her last few years, when she really required help, we had made peace.

I had willingly stood between my mother and her greatest fear: going to a nursing home. I had agonized whether I would be able to finish the task. We had not told her about David and AIDS, but she knew that her grandson had some kind of blood disease. My mother had accepted the fact that he was my primary concern.

Fate had not forced me to make an impossible decision, and my mother had died peacefully at home, as she had wished so fervently. She had not been well, a week earlier, when I had bid her good-bye before leaving for California. I will always wonder whether my—temporary—absence had given her license to die.

Services for my Mom were held at the Riverside Memorial Chapel, where we had gathered for my father 41 years earlier. At the time, my mother, my sister and I had been completely traumatized by my father's untimely death, a short three years after we had finally been reunited in New York after a six year long separation. My mother's funeral was much easier. I proudly looked at my parents' two sons-in-law, four grandchildren, and twin great-granddaughters. Life had fulfilled some of its promises. My family had survived the Holocaust and had found a new home in America. Perhaps there would be a cure for AIDS before I had to give up my son! I looked at him standing up front, delivering his eulogy:

> "To me, it's very appropriate that Greta Garbo and my Omi should have died so close to one another—you see, as a child I sometimes thought they were the same or at least similar people. Both were so glamorous, elegant and beautiful.
>
> I have often stared at the pastel picture of my grandmother that hangs in her foyer and thought, how beautiful.
>
> Of course, Omi wasn't really like Greta Garbo—she was much more fun. I have so many memories of wonderful times together.
>
> Like going hiking in the Swiss Alps (which were actually her furniture in the living room in her house in Forest Hills), and picnicking in a make-shift tent under the coffee table.
>
> Or going to see such movies as "That Darn Cat," and "Its a Mad Mad Mad Mad World." Some of the first movies I really remember.
>
> Later, our tastes matured (it seemed together) and we saw Fellini and Bergman, always followed by lively and adult conversation. And the museums, musicals and music. Omi didn't like to talk while we sat in her living room listening intently to the classical music…
>
> Some of my strongest memories of Omi have to do with walking—we literally used to run from one side of Manhattan to the other. My little eight or twelve-year old legs had to work hard to keep up with her. "Walking keeps me young," she used to say.
>
> Ironically it was from the time her medical problems prevented her from walking that I date her decline.

Still, our relationship was so simple and so good that even when we didn't go out as much, or later go out at all, we had a great time together. There was always Scrabble—I never could quite beat her until very recently.

Last July, on my way to Europe—a trip largely taken [with my mother] to explore our Belgian past, I stopped in New York, mainly to see Omi.

On this particular visit Judy, Ana and Naomi were there with me. As we sat around the table with our take-out Chinese food—I had a revelation. All of us are born with an inner spirit that basically remains the same and is with us throughout our entire lives. Ana and Naomi have theirs—and Omi has hers. The intellect and circumstances change, but the core remains the same. Omi, diminished as she was, still had her essence.

Now that Omi is gone, perhaps a little of her spirit lives on in those who loved her.

I want to thank my mom and dad for seeing that she was so well cared for.

After the relief of having shepherded my mom safely through her old age lifted, I started missing her. I could appreciate what she had taught me: the ability to think for myself, to stand up for what I believed in, and most of all to persevere when life seemed bleak.

David and I were back in California for his birthday on February 19th. When my children had been small, and I kissed them goodnight on their birthday, we took a fantasy trip to a magic star that held all the things they could wish for. Now my sentimental son wanted me to tell him about the star for 35-year olds. I really only had one wish for him—a magic bullet to shield him from AIDS, though for good measure his star was bathed in perpetual sunshine, peopled with handsome men, and stocked with gourmet food, designer clothes, and other treats.

My good wishes started to stick in my throat. By now David's T-cells were below 100.

"It does not matter," I said. "People live 'forever' without any T cells. It is how one feels that counts. Your P24"—an indicator of virus load—"is still negative, and new drugs are coming down the pipeline."

I knew that I was lying. I was worried sick. The sons and daughters of the mothers in my support group were getting sick and dying.

The 1991 birthday party was my swan song at 902 Haight. Keith Potter had moved out in 1989. Paying the entire rent had become a struggle, and David decided to look for smaller, cheaper quarters. We went apartment shopping. The dog and the need for a garage were a hindrance, but David finally found a small one bedroom, on Seventeenth Street, in San Francisco's Mission District. Until this day I don't know whether the deciding factor for David was the apartment or his new landlord.

In New York I had had to empty my mom's apartment. Medals should be bestowed on those who sort out someone else's life-long debris. Digging through other people's possessions is an intrusion into their souls, their dreams, defeats, secrets, messes, and trivialities.

My mother actually had been restrained about accumulating flotsam. Still, there were dozens of ugly nylon shifts that she would have shunned in her more with-it days, dozens of candles, cartons of milk powder to nourish her during an atomic attack, and similar useless "stuff." There were lots of books, china, photographs, letters, and other mementos that she had miraculously shepherded through World War II or collected since.

The letters were in a haphazard jumble. I skimmed them all, discovering that she had been more loving than I had given her credit for. Some missives recalled the horrors of World War II. One postcard, dating from 1939, read in part: "The nightmare even becomes more real when one puts it into concrete words." This shocking reminder of those schizophrenic times could have been written about AIDS.

Two months after my mother's death, Judy gave birth to Sean, her third child. Like his sisters, he was born at St. Vincent's Hospital, where so many of the children of my Mothers' Group had died of AIDS. Life was such a mixed bag!

A month after Sean's birth, David and his friends left for a bicycle trip in Italy. He was flying through New York and we were to meet him at Kennedy. David's diary records his adventures:

"European trip May 10–28, 1991:

Last night was hectic…I was finished [packing] by midnight…I only slept for a little more than five hours…now 8:20 AM we are taxiing already. I feel calm, happy (not haapppy-happy) and energetic.

"I am so excited that I'm going to meet Sean—almost, or rally as excited as about the trip. Happy also to be seeing the rest of the family. The whole trip is also very wonderful sounding and feeling."

David landed in Zurich, and visited with distant relatives, including my father's 85-year old cousin: "Walter, wonderful to meet…history comes more to life talking with him…"

Two days later David took the train to Chiusi in Tuscany:

"I am in the middle of the most exciting, beautiful train ride of my life. At 6:24 AM we pulled out of Zurich. The hills and lakes are shrouded in a lacy, delicate mist...at 7:30 the sun breaks through and I glimpse the snow capped and craggy mountains...

"By my AZT clock I have been up six hours...in a way that seems a long time, in a way not long enough...excited about seeing the boys [his San Francisco friends]... I'm having a fantastic time...Arrived in Chiusi at 4:52 PM, right on time. Everybody was there...it's wonderful to see them."

The group bicycled up and down hills, photographing each other, feasting on art and wonderful food as they went along. "Incredible dinner last night," David recorded, "lasted over four hours: Bruschetta, crostini misti, gnochetti with pesto, pici with Bolognese, scottigia, veal, vinsanto, passito, etc."

"Wednesday...Another wonderful day, although at this moment am pretty beat...[there was] thunder and lightning on the tortuous hill coming up to Montalino..."

David smiled at us from the eight rolls of film he brought back, and the tour company used his picture in their 1992 catalog.

"Was a great trip," he wrote in the diary on the return flight. "Really was happy most of the time. Many 'perfect moments.'"

Then AIDS and reality intruded: "Still don't know about [going on] disability or how to handle medical treatment. I am looking forward to Liza, Joseph, my new picture, play! I want to make a will, arrange photos."

During his return trip David even questioned his relationship with Margie, his beloved therapist, and with his mother.

"Is therapy addictive?" he writes. "Is Mom too special and in the way of other relationships? Does that hold for Margie too?"

◆   ◆   ◆

New mothers kept coming to our group at a rate of 35 to 40 a year. By now the group was nationally known and served as a model for groups in other cities. Sessions, as always, were a mixed blessing. I needed the camaraderie, the feeling of being connected. I participated, shared my joys and fears, and yet.... Why was AIDS still universally fatal ten years after it had emerged? I could not stand all those deaths and memorials. Why did I go to group? Was it to prepare for the terrible times that lay ahead? Did I believe that vicarious suffering protected my son?

One evening in 1990, Blanche Mednick, a 42-year old elementary school teacher, showed up. Initially she was reserved and distant. Incredible sadness filled her big brown eyes, and one could sense a deep inner hurt, yet she rarely expressed her anger—or even her anguish—openly.

Pain and loneliness were, however, only one aspect of Blanche's personality. She always spoke with profound compassion, and intelligence, and had a wonderful sense of humor. I loved the way she poked fun at herself.

Blanche came to the group because a contaminated needle had infected her 24-year old son, Brian, a former drug-user. Brian's HIV-status had only been diagnosed a few months earlier, and he still was in denial.

Brian was a child of the streets. Early in life he had started to rely on himself. He was proud of his Italian heritage, and his most cherished possession was a heavy gold bracelet adorned with weighty medals.

Blanche's family had been poor and dysfunctional. She was convinced that many of her own difficulties stemmed from having grown up on welfare. As a single mother, Blanche was determined to provide Brian with what she had lacked.

"Not being on welfare was my single, overriding goal," she recalled. "At the time it was more important to me than nursing Brian or staying home with him. Naively, I believed that if I paid my bills, he would pay his bills, that if I went to school, he would want to become a scholar, that if I read and wrote poetry, he would love books."

For many years this approach had worked. Brian was a lovable child. He enchanted everyone he met. He drew well, wrote, and was a whiz at languages.

"When he was four," Blanche recalled, "I met Jerry. He and Brian established a loving relationship, and for ten days the three of us went off to Greece. Brian picked up Greek much more rapidly than Jerry or I did." Soon the child could buy pretzels and fruit from the kiosks on the islands.

Then things had started to go wrong. When Brian was twelve, Blanche discovered that he was smoking pot. "I was very young and inexperienced," she recalled, "and trusted the establishment so implicitly that I went the therapeutic route. When the therapy did not work, and Brian began to spend more time on the streets, Blanche took him to Juvenile Court—there she took out a petition declaring him a delinquent. Brian then agreed to finish school if he could live in a foster set-up with a a friend's foster father. Blanche agreed. This didn't work either and Blanche suspected the foster father of being a pedophile, but couldn't prove it.

Most mothers blame themselves for their children's problems. As Blanche recalled, "It took me a long time to understand that Brian and I were very different. I thrive on solitude; he could not stand being by himself. Some of Brian's difficulties had nothing to do with me. Many of his father's relatives were manic-depressives. Brian was a hyperactive child, suffering from a chemical dependency factor. I am convinced that if drugs had been legalized and clean needles available, my son would not have been infected."

Blanche believed that all mothers, but especially those belonging to our group, had an innate "magic power." She figured that if her own "magic" could not save her child, he surely would be saved by the combined "magic" of the group.

Eventually Blanche realized that we could not cure Brian, but she experienced a different sort of magic. She responded to the kindness and compassion of the group and opened up. And she made a true friend.

Rhea and Blanche were opposites and complementary. Blanche was a loner, Rhea a social magnet. Blanche was depressive, Rhea always smiled. Their life experience, however, had been remarkably alike. Both grew up in the sixties and were single mothers. Their sons took pride in the Italian heritage of their absentee fathers.

The affinity of the mothers did not extend to their children. Adam was gay and sophisticated. Brian was heterosexual and "macho." Adam wished that his mother had a beeper and could respond to his every real and imagined need. Brian was distant, often disappearing for months. He still rejected his intellectual, sensitive mother. Adam explored every medical alternative, Brian refused to acknowledge that there was anything wrong with him. For a long time, he would not take any of the anti-viral medications that retarded the progression of AIDS.

Slowly, however, Blanche and her son reestablished the bond that had united them during Brian's early childhood. She paid heavily for regaining Brian and immersing herself into his care. Her second husband started drinking, vandalized their home, and left.

The summer of 1991 was mercifully uneventful. Ernest and I enjoyed our cottage in Maine. David managed to have another week's vacation and spent it with Judy and her family on the Cape. When October rolled around, I journeyed to San Francisco.

David's new apartment was too small for me to stay at comfortably for more than a few days. My son, however, had located quarters that I could sublet whenever the tenant, a dancer, was on tour. The minute David saw the place he knew that I would love it.

He was right. The aerie-like loft was carved out of the attic of an old Victorian house, the birthplace of my 75-year-old landlady. Her mother had already transformed the backyard into an Eden of tall trees, plants, cacti, flowers, and brick walks. A small fountain gurgled continuously. I climbed to my third floor "tree house" via an outdoor staircase. I was short-winded when I got to the top, but was enchanted by the San Francisco back yards that surrounded me. All was quiet, except for an occasional dog bark cascading around the neighborhood.

David usually took the bus to work. When I was in town, I went to his house at eight AM, loaded Liza in the car and drove to AT & T, so that David would be less late than usual. After dropping David off, Liza and I walked in Golden Gate Park. On the way home, I stopped at my friend the butcher for some unusual cut of meat or other delicacy. "Your lucky son," the butcher used to tease. I spent the day writing and cooking, interrupted by numerous calls from my son.

At five-thirty I picked David up at work. Our routine was punctuated by doctors' appointments, pentamidine treatments, acupuncture, small dinner parties, psychotherapy, acting classes, support group sessions, hassles with insurance companies, and other grim reminders that the virus was ticking away in David's body.

My visits, I hoped, provided David with some relief from everyday stresses and strains, including his job at AT & T. During the eight years he worked there he often hated it.

Perhaps his discontent was a manifestation of dealing with a fatal illness; perhaps he felt trapped. Perhaps it was the basic mismatch of David's creative talents and a humdrum job. The phone company, however, was a safety net, paid David's medical bills, offered many perks, and provided him with a normal, structured existence. I foresaw years of him being unemployed and ill and wanted to postpone that heartache for both him and me. Circumstances worked out differently. By the time the illness overtook him, David was fully employed. He even had found himself another job at AT & T and was excited about his future there.

The cruelest aspect of AIDS was its total unpredictability. The disease had more ways of killing its prey than Hercules' nine-headed hydra: *pneumocystis* pneumonia, toxoplasmosis, KS, tuberculosis, leukemias, lymphomas, *cytomegalovirus* (CMV), *cryptospirosis…*

Death, however, is not what terrifies most patients. It is the uncontrollable diarrhea, the incontinence, the blindness, the dementia, the neuropathies, the emaciation, the impotence, the inability to walk, the gradual loss of control and function.

In people with a malfunctioning immune system, the cytomegalovirus (CMV) commonly destroyed the retina of the eye. Provided it was diagnosed early, two nasty drugs administered by continuous IV drip could arrest this deterioration. Regular eye examinations were thus part of routine AIDS care.

My son was more terrified of loosing his eyesight than of most other opportunistic infections. He postponed visits to Dr. N., an AIDS eye specialist, until I was in town, or he could marshal a friend to come with him. Before each visit David would be hysterical Fortunately, David's retinas remained clear as bells.

During the three years David was his patient, Dr. N., an enthusiastic amateur photographer, moved his office from his modest quarters to very elegant digs, paid for by his thriving AIDS practice. Portraits of AIDS patients, with their birth and death dates, lined his examining room! I still regret not having confronted the doctor with the insensitivity of his photo exhibit.

I disliked Dr. N. intensely, even more so when I realized that his diagnostic equipment was antiquated and in no way matched the elegance of the furniture. Fortunately, David found a more compassionate ophthalmologist who entered him in a drug trial designed to prevent visual damage. My son was somewhat reassured, though it meant an additional six pills a day.

Kaposi's sarcoma, the disfiguring red skin cancer, a dead give-away of AIDS, was also universally despised. Early in its course KS could also be treated quite successfully with radiation or chemotherapy.

David hated the emaciation that accompanied the late stages of AIDS. Often when we walked down the street, he would point out somebody who clearly suffered from AIDS-induced wasting syndrome. Fortunately, I could often think of someone who had lost a tremendous amount of weight and then regained it. "Remember," I told him, "when Dave Nelson had TB he lost 30 pounds, which he put back on quickly when his tuberculosis was under control."

David fortunately had not lost any weight. He and his friends joked about their "whale-like girth." David joined Weight Watchers, lost twenty pounds, and was as svelte and youthful looking as ever.

7

TWILIGHT

I greeted 1992 with my customary wish: Let me not be worse off next year than I am now. But my apprehension was escalating, and David too was feeling more desperate and anxious. Back in 1983, when he first suspected that he was a carrier, he had told himself that he had ten years before he would develop overt disease. By then, he figured, there certainly would be a cure. Now, a decade later, the AIDS virus was still calling the shots.

One sign of David's growing anxiety was the telephone. Before HIV we talked once or twice a week, then several times a week, then once or twice daily. There were also cards and letters.

January 1992

Sweetie-pie,

I have a wonderful card for you, but may not be able to find it on my messy desk before I mail this letter…

I thought about our conversation last night. I am sorry that you are depressed. It is only surprising that you are not depressed more often. Your question: "what have I to look forward to?" kept echoing in my mind.

Though your time frame may be different, eventually we all must die. Last week, seeing "Dancing at Lughansa" on Broadway, I told Dad that I wish I wouldn't wake up tomorrow. I know that I will have to face more surgery for my arthritis. If I live too long I will be blind (glaucoma) and most of all there always is the possibility of you getting sick.

But, though part of me wants "out" another part of me knows that I can't do that to those who love me so very much: Ana, Naomi, Judy, you, or Daddy.

And then there are the good times that lie ahead: my little apartment in San Francisco, spending some weeks with you, the sun in Hawaii, the next piece of chocolate, another book sale.

As long as one breathes life is a mixed bag…

You have known about, and struggled with, HIV for so very long. You have had your emotional ups and downs dealing with it. Trust yourself—you'll continue to triumph.

I saw the Wizard of Oz with the girls. Remember what the Wiz said to the tin man after he got his heart? "Now you have a heart; it is there to be broken." Or later: "It is not how many people love you that counts, but how many people you love..." I am still glad that my heart is big, even though it gets sad often.

Oh well! I am looking forward to talking to you in 45 minutes, and going to Hawaii, [David's 1992 birthday present] and spending four weeks with you in February, and then again, and again and again.

At the end of February that year the two of us journeyed to Kauai. Our condo had two lanais, one facing the ocean, the other the cliffs of the Napali coast. We swam, hiked and laughed. David was feeling well and looked smashing. I can still see the smile on his face as he luxuriated in the Jacuzzi or the sparkle in his eye when he sipped champagne. Why was I so keyed up then? Why could I not forget about this damned disease?

Ever since his success in *Gays in Our Lives* David had wanted to be in another play. In the spring of 1992 he auditioned at the Alameda Play House and snagged the role of stage manager in *Enter Laughing*. David was delighted. He drove the 20 miles to Alameda for endless rehearsals and three weekly performances in spite of a full time job, his cumbersome medical care, and his regular workouts at the gym. David thrived on the acting, and at each performance his many friends enlarged the audience. I was in California for one of my periodic visits, and enjoyed seeing my son the actor. I wondered whether David's pleasure in performing was worth the additional strain. I kept my mouth shut.

There was talk of immuno-modulation, e.g. the rebuilding of a severely impaired immune system. Patients with advanced AIDS were transfused with white blood cells harvested from healthier HIV-positive patients. David thought that Stewart Mittler, his friend from Brandeis, might be a likely donor.

While waiting for a major breakthrough, it turned out that old-fashioned sulfa drugs were a more effective prophylaxis against *pneumocystis* than aerosol pentamidine. Why had it taken doctors so long to figure that out? Conant felt that David should switch to sulfa drugs because he had used pentamidine for such a long time that by now he might harbor a pentamidine-resistant strain of *pneumocystis*.

The trouble was that David was severely allergic to sulfa drugs. Since these allergies were common, Conant was working on a desensitization technique. In this scheme patients were to take ever-increasing amounts of sulfa for a period of ten days.

David's drug reaction to the sulfa started after day five. He developed a low-grade fever a few hours after taking the drug. He was not deterred. He took aspirin, went to work, performed in Alameda and stayed up late.

In honor of my visit, David took a day off from AT & T. We had planned to drive to Mendocino, the old fishing port we had loved in 1977 during our first trip up the North Coast. The Loebls are a stubborn lot. In spite of David's increasingly severe drug reaction we started for Mendocino, equipped with sulfa drugs, aspirin and cortisone. The aspirin was meant to control the fever, the cortisone the drug reaction. David's fever was getting higher. We kept calling Conant's office to ask for advice. "Carry on," they said, "increase the cortisone."

David drove, at his usual fast clip, the thermometer sticking out of his mouth. The fever came and went. He developed a rash. We checked into our motel in Mendocino. After David took a cold shower, the fever dropped. I went to the front desk and asked for both the location of the closest hospital and of the best restaurant in town! Did the manager think his guests needed a loony bin?

Mendocino was as good as we remembered it, reminding David of Provincetown, me of Maine. The meal at Mendocino's best restaurant was truly great, but I was sick with anxiety and had a hard time swallowing the rosemary-perfumed roast leg of lamb with "pubescent" vegetables and gratinéed potatoes.

David's rash kept spreading. He was as red as a boiled lobster. We returned to San Francisco. I broke the mercury thermometer as I was shaking it down. We bought another one. David woke me in the middle of the night. His fever was above 104°. I dumped him into an ice-cold bath. The shock of the cold water was almost unendurable. David shivered and his teeth chattered wildly. The fever broke, but that was the end of the sulfa. David was the one failure in Conant's otherwise successful study.

The failure, however, also undermined our faith in pentamadine. To convince him to enter in the study, Conant had explained that pentamadine prophylaxis was only 80% effective.

There was other bad news. The big swollen lymph gland in his neck, which David believed manufactured "good" helper (T_8) cells, had disappeared.

◆   ◆   ◆

In August the entire family spent a week with Ernest and me in Maine. Our cottage was a bit small for the eight of us, but I loved having my entire brood under one roof, even though there were some tensions. We were a typical 1960's family, and our children felt entitled to complain—a lot—about how we had brought them up. I always imagined that other parents did better, but maybe they too were frustrated.

One welcome visitor to Maine that summer was Robert Driscoll, a friend of David's from business school. Robert, like David, was still looking for an "ideal" partner. That year David had several new boyfriends, but in each case AIDS interfered with a long-term commitment. Jerry, the first of the series, was very much smitten with my son. Actually the two might have been a good match. Both came from middle-class Jewish homes, both were smart, good looking, athletic and shared many interests. Jerry, however, was so terrified of my son's HIV-status that David called it quits. If I had been Jerry's mother I would have been relieved by his caution. As it was, I was bitter on my son's behalf, and the incident clearly indicated how many doors this wretched disease was slamming shut.

Joe, David's second potential boyfriend, was a very handsome intellectual lightweight. He too was much taken with my son, but Joe rekindled the nasty streak that had marred many of David's childhood friendships. David exploited Joe's willingness to do chores. My son's San Francisco family was relieved when Joe got his walking papers.

David had met Rick, an airline steward, at a dance in New York. During the fall of 1992, the two spent a few days in Mexico, and Rick became passionately committed to David, showering him with attention. Though David liked Rick, he felt that the emotional burden he was already carrying kept him from becoming intensely involved.

My aerie on Sanchez Street was available in early November, and I flew out to California on Election Day, having cast my vote for Clinton in New York earlier. David had been a Democratic district captain and was invited to a victory party. "I never voted for anyone I cared for before," David told me. His enthusiasm was contagious. We went to the celebration, attended by Barbara Boxer, the newly elected senator from California. We walked home through star-studded San Francisco, imagining that our handsome baby-boomer president would do for AIDS and for gays what the Republicans had neglected.

I always had well-developed extrasensory perception. I often know who is on the phone before I pick it up, and answer people's questions before they have been asked. This bond was especially strong with my son. Once, when I chimed in on one of his inner conversations he angrily called me a circus clown. I couldn't help my increasing despondence about David's health, though there was no overt sign that he was getting worse. He still looked radiant, and even now, as I look at the photographs from December 1992, he smiles in every picture. Though I tried to be as positive as I could about AIDS, David noted that I had become less upbeat and told me so. I now wonder whether I abandoned my son before his time was up?

8

ARMAGEDDON

Sometimes the Mothers' Group perked along quite peacefully. At others, when many of our children were very ill, or when there were several deaths, the going was rough. So it was in the second half of 1992.

Blanche had lost her son, Brian, that July. Until April of that year, Brian had done well. He had held several part-time jobs, rented an apartment of his own, and seemed "clean." He had found a woman he wanted to marry, started to nest and proudly told his mother of his culinary feats. At his fiancée's request he had become a Roman Catholic, and had invited Blanche and Rhea to his First Communion.

Brian's future in-laws had been planning an elaborate May wedding. Two months before the event, Eleanor, his bride-to-be, had succumbed to her own manic-depressive illness. Brian had been forced to commit her to St. Vincent's psychiatric ward. He was emotionally incapable of living on his own, or caring for his fiancée. Within a month of Eleanor's hospitalization he had returned to drugs. When Brian had not answered his phone, a worried Eleanor had asked her father to check their apartment. Brian had overdosed and was unconscious. An ambulance took him to Cabrini Hospital, where they put him on a respirator.

At the hospital Brian hovered between life and death. Blanche was constantly at his bedside, communicating with him in spite of the respirator. Sometimes they cried together, sometimes they were angry at each other, sometimes they were at peace, "pretending," as Blanche told us, "that this was not the end."

Within weeks after he arrived at Cabrini, the AIDS virus took over Brian's body. He suffered from pneumonia, gall bladder failure, tuberculosis, candida, and other opportunistic infections, but he didn't die. Blanche implored the hospital to shut off the respirator. Because this was a Catholic institution, they refused. Finally the hospital agreed to let Blanche ask Brian to blink twice if he wished life-support to cease. Brian died on July 7, 69 days after his admission.

◆　　　◆　　　◆

The group had gotten to know Rhea's son, Adam Balzano, well. In spite of AIDS, Adam had obtained a scholarship to New York University's film school, earning an A in all his courses. A documentary about the Mothers' Group was to be his thesis. During the Fall of 1992 he had interviewed some of us and filmed several group sessions. We all felt proud of him.

In November, long before the film was finished, Adam started to fail. He had persistent headaches, diarrhea, coughed, lost weight, and ran a fever. A CT of the brain showed a mass. For weeks Adam's physicians were mystified. Eventually they diagnosed tuberculosis. Under the circumstances, that was good news. Most often, TB is treatable. Still, Adam was furious about having to battle yet another opportunistic infection.

"I went to see Dr. Berkowitz," Rhea told us the following week. "I asked him whether this might be Adam's last Thanksgiving. I wanted him to deny it, but he didn't. I know that I must be prepared to lose Adam, but I just can't face that possibility." For once, even Rhea cried.

Thanksgiving was even worse than Rhea had foreseen. She had invited her mother, who had not seen Adam since August.

"I had warned her that Adam looked so thin that he was almost transparent. So she knew what to expect. Nevertheless, when she saw him she said, 'This is not my Adam.'"

Grandma was terrified by Adam's cough, and asked Rhea for separate dishes. "I was going to argue," Rhea told the group, "but Adam took his grandmother in stride. 'Give her different dishes, Mom, but not the good ones,' he said."

"Adam is so tired of being ill." Rhea told us. "Now he really looks like he has AIDS. Last night he wet his bed for the first time. That was very upsetting to both of us."

"I really start to envy others," Rhea said bitterly on another occasion, "even people I like. When I see young couples hugging, kissing and having a good time I get furious and resentful. Why should Adam be cheated of all that. Why him?"

In spite of his deteriorating health, Rhea and Adam were planning to fly to Maui in January. Rhea was scared to death of the trip, but like the rest of us, tried to grant her son's every wish.

"We have friends in Maui," Rhea explained bravely. "Adam has visited them before. They have a little baby boy Adam, named for my Adam. He wants to meet his namesake."

This, however, was not the trip's sole purpose. Adam wanted to pick the spot at which his mother was to scatter his ashes.

I looked at Rhea and the other women in the group. I felt ill. Was I hearing right? How could we calmly discuss our children's funerals? Was this my life? When would I wake up from this nightmare?

Mind-boggling as these conversations were, it was not even appropriate to avoid them. We knew how guilty our children felt for causing us such pain. We had to let them know that we would be "all right" after it was all over!

Rhea continued: "Adam and I talk a lot about dying, but I really don't know how he feels about it. With Adam it is always theatrical. He never cries, I cry."A week later Rhea sounded a bit more cheerful

"We went to see Berkowitz today and he made us feel better," she told us. "The doctor had pointed out that a year ago Adam had had a brain lesion and today he just had a very minor neurological impairment." Berkowitz had said that Adam could be better, but that he could also be much worse. Still, Rhea assured us, Berkowitz was encouraged by Adam's response to the TB medication and the absence of fever.

I visited Adam with some homemade pesto a few days before the Maui trip. He savored a big plate full of spaghetti with pesto like a seasoned gourmet. "You have to give my mother your recipe," he insisted. "She does not know how to make pesto."

Adam was tethered to an IV drip and had trouble walking across the room. He was nevertheless most excited about the Hawaii trip. He had used his frequent flyer miles to upgrade their airline tickets. "Mom and I have never flown first class," he explained.

I could hardly hold back my tears. "This whole shitty disease is so crazy-making," I told myself. "Here is this young, talented man, full of plans and loving life. He is not even 30 years old and he is about to die, while I with all my aches and pains, have years to live.!"

Rhea had checked out the AIDS services on Maui, located a support group for herself, and arranged for wheelchairs at every airport.

"Imagine—Maui's AIDS support group meets on Tuesday nights', just like ours," Rhea told us before she left.

◆   ◆   ◆

Beryl Aaron had joined our group in 1991, when her son, Howard, had tested positive for HIV. Like Blanche, Beryl had a dry, self-deprecating sense of humor, and whenever she came to group we laughed. Beryl was a high-level executive, jet-setted across the country, had a fancy car, a new mink coat, and dated men in distant cities. She brought us a glimpse of a more glamorous world than that of the hospital corridors and doctors' offices that were our usual fare.

In spite of all that glitter, Beryl was as frightened as the rest of us, feeling as if a "sharp sword" was constantly hanging over her head." Howard was not her only problem. Beryl came from a strict Syrian Jewish Community in Brooklyn in which women stayed at home. A dozen years earlier she had ruffled tradition by divorcing her alcoholic husband, going to work and making a success of it. Such "unseemly behavior" made her an outcast. Even her brother no longer spoke to her. This did not deter Beryl. When Howard "came out," she stood by him, as well as by Ellen, her freethinking, sexually liberated daughter.

One evening Beryl told the group about a party she had attended with her latest beau.

"The hosts had arranged for a fortune teller. As a dare I too had my cards read. The fortuneteller said that I had two children and she proceeded to tell me lot of good stuff about Ellen, my daughter.

"Then the fortuneteller's face changed. 'I see something terrible happening to your son this September. He is ill, and his disease is taking a turn for the worse. He is going to die.'

"I was terrified." Beryl continued. "The fortuneteller could not possible know that Howard is HIV positive!"

Beryl's experience was not unique. Another one of our mothers, Priscilla Reed, was haunted by such a prediction.

It was hard to believe that Priscilla was a grandmother—the full-time custodian of her seven-year-old grandson, Noah.

Priscilla was twenty when she married her childhood sweetheart, and not much older when she had her own two children, Rob and Cathleen. The Reeds led a pleasant, uneventful life in the suburbs. Priscilla finished college, majoring in music and education. When she was widowed, she had to bring up her children as a single parent.

The strain did not ease after the children were grown. Cathleen married, had a son and started drugging. Soon thereafter, Michael, her husband left. Cathleen's life was so unstable that, at Rob's urging, Priscilla eventually assumed legal guardianship of Noah, her grandson. Priscilla's teaching job and Rob's small landscape business paid for two apartments, private school for Noah, a full-time babysitter, clothes, toys and food.

Then Rob, unaware that he was HIV positive, developed full-blown AIDS. There was no health insurance. Rob struggled with nausea, weight loss, vomiting, and diarrhea. He raged at his sister and his disease. Rob did not believe in mainstream medicine and refused to see a doctor, saying "Everybody with AIDS dies no matter what."

At home, Priscilla kept up a brave front, but at the Mothers' Group her pain flowed freely and her fears enveloped us all.

The evening Beryl told the group about her Tarot reading, Priscilla told us about her own burden. "Years ago, I regularly consulted an astrologer. I asked her many questions about my grandson. One day I noticed that the medium became very agitated and frightened when she looked at my horoscope.

"She did not want to tell me what she saw, but I insisted. Eventually she told me that she foresaw a major change in Noah's life when he turned eight. I figured that Cathleen might overdose, or that I might get sick, or that Michael, Cathleen's ex, would come back and make trouble about custody…. In any case, the event was far in the future, and I forgot about it." Priscilla's voice broke as she added, "The other day I suddenly remembered this prediction and now I can't forget it. Noah is going to be eight years old in February…."

Like her son, Priscilla shunned conventional medicine. They battled Rob's symptoms with herbs and home remedies. One evening Susan Katz pointed out that the two of them colluded in their denial of AIDS. "Rob is suffering even more than he needs to," Susan said. "You must acknowledge AIDS. Not availing yourself of whatever medical help is available does not help Rob."

Instead of answering, Priscilla said, "I sometimes wonder whether I am so terrified about Rob's disease because he helps me care for Noah."

One evening in early January, 1993, Priscilla arrived at the meeting more agitated than usual. "Last week Cathleen's ex called and thanked me for taking care of his son. I was taken aback. Never before had he expressed any gratitude. Then he asked whether he could come and visit. Cathleen had cautioned me not to allow him near Noah or even to send him photographs. She was afraid that Michael might kidnap the boy."

"I wondered whether Cathleen's concern was justified or was an expression of her own paranoia," Priscilla said. "I did not want to deprive Noah of a relationship he is entitled to.

"To help me sort things out, I went to consult a friend of mine—a child psychiatrist who lives in the Bronx. My appointment was in the late afternoon, and since the Bronx is not the safest place in the world, Rob wanted to come along to protect me. He kept insisting, but he had a doctor's appointment, which I did not want him to break, so I prevailed.

"Actually we all had been in a relatively happy frame of mind. It was Friday and I had promised to take Rob and Noah out for dinner."

Before driving to the Bronx for her appointment, Priscilla had gone to the bank to get money for the outing.

"As I was driving back to Manhattan via the Willis Avenue Bridge," Priscilla continued, "I stopped for a red light. Suddenly one guy blocked the front of my car, and another shattered my car window. I didn't know whether the two had come to kill me, or what…I stepped on the gas, hard. When I finally regained my balance I noticed that my big black leather bag was missing from the front seat. It held all my papers, my bankcard, my appointment book, the money we were going to eat out with. The whole thing was so incredibly fast….

"When I got home I had to tell Rob. He went off the deep end. He kept saying that he knew that it was going to happen. Then he started cursing his sister. 'S-H-I-T C-A-T,' he kept screaming over and over again. He spelled the words out so that Noah would not understand. He pummeled the walls with his fists. He went on and on.

"Then he said that he would kill himself. I heard him retch, cough and run to the bathroom all night. He would not talk to me, and the next morning he left. He has not called me since and doesn't answer his phone.

"I can't stand it when he rejects me like that. I plead and refuse to leave him alone. I always want to do something for him, help him beat the disease. I go to the store and buy papaya juice or something else which might make him feel better. I am so vulnerable right now. Both my children are in such danger. I may lose them both by next year."

"Rob is not angry at you," Alice said. "He is frustrated by the disease, by his inability to protect you from the vandals, by his dependency, by his fear."

"Priscilla, "Susan Katz said, "I want you to give Rob his space now. You may know what therapists call the law of the 'distancer and the pursuer.' The two of you are totally intertwined; you pursue Rob, and he runs away. Such an intense relationship is appropriate for a baby, not for a grown man. This bond was bound to snap. I guarantee you that the sooner you let Rob go, the sooner he will come back."

◆   ◆   ◆

One evening during this terrible autumn, Lucy showed up. She was tall and thin like a model. Her long, wavy hair made her look almost like a teenager, though she too told us that she was a grandmother.

Lucy came from an Italian family, but her childhood home had none of the legendary warmth. "I really was a deprived child. My parents never, never hugged or kissed me. They taught me pain and fear." It took Lucy more than forty years to come to terms with her anguish and have some faith in life.

At sixteen, to get away from home, Lucy married the first available man. In rapid succession, she gave birth to two boys, John and Philip. Married life was no better for Lucy than her childhood had been. There was no money for food, let alone for the drugs and alcohol that were part of the family fare. Somehow Lucy and her two sons survived. After eleven years of abuse, she left her husband.

Slowly Lucy made a life for herself, eventually meeting Walter, who loved her in spite of her self-contempt. Alcohol and drug abuse were, however, deeply ingrained in her sons' life-style. Lucy believed that now John was finally "clean and dry", but Philip was not. She had come to the group because during one of his many prison sojourns Philip had tested positive for the AIDS virus.

During her first evening at the group, Lucy had described herself as being "totally crazy," because Philip was about to be released from Riker's Island prison.

"I am not preparing for it. When he was picked up last June he was very sick—he had a kidney infection, mites, and the blood vessels in his arms were as thick as ropes. After he was picked up, they cleaned him up in prison. They offered rehab, but he refused. He went back to live on the street then, and he is going to do the same now. On the street he'll go fast."

"How old is Philip?" Priscilla asked. "Twenty-five," Lucy answered. "Oh God," Priscilla cried out. "A baby, we are losing babies."

The following week Priscilla apologized to the entire group for having been too outspoken.

Addressing Lucy, she said, "I am so glad to see you here tonight. I thought you might never come back. Last week I let out all my raw anger. All these babies who are going to die…"

Lucy did not need any apologies. "You gave me a gift. I finally could cry. Usually I only feel terrified, guilty and numb, but still unable to cry. I need to cry so badly that I sometimes rent a sad movie. Even then I don't always manage.

"When you talked about 'our babies dying,' I did cry. Then I told myself how wonderful. I've found a place where I can cry. I can go there every Tuesday and cry."

Deane told Priscilla not to be apologetic about what she said. "Where else can you let it all out?" she asked. Priscilla had relaxed, but now she tensed up again.

"How are you standing it? I look around me here, and everybody else seems resigned and I am fighting this disease as if I were a wild horse, I am kicking my hooves. I know that I have to knuckle under eventually, but I don't want to give up now."

"Nobody is resigned," Alice said. "Sometimes we think we are resigned, but that is when 'they' are holding their own. Last time I visited Gilbert in San Francisco, he was so sick that I thought I would come home with his ashes. But when I saw him I wanted him to live…and thank God he got better. He came home for Christmas and we had a wonderful visit, the best time we've had in a long while. You are wrong. No mother here gives up. We all fight like hell."

Emily turned to Priscilla: "Don't hold back your pain. You help us, you express what we feel, we all hurt so terribly…."

Lucy talked some more about Philip.

"I wish that I could take care of him, nurse him, He was born when I was 17. I may not have been the best mother. I should have been more loving, warmer. But how could I give him warmth when I was a needy kid myself? When Philip was ten years old, his father was killed in a motorcycle accident. When Philip was 17 he gave up on life. He was hooked on drugs and it has been hell ever since." Lucy continued:

"When Philip is in prison I am OK. Now that he is about to be released I worry and I hate myself for worrying. Philip has my unlisted phone number, but not my address. I am afraid he'll find my house. I constantly look over my shoulder when I leave my house. I wonder whether he is there, watching and waiting…I hate answering my telephone…Philip is so good at twisting my heart. The other day he told me that he is 'going to see his Dad soon.' "I realize that I must ignore such tactics," she continued, "but knowing that Philip is HIV-positive makes it harder. He will die! I feel I haven't even earned the right to grieve. I know that some day I'll have to make amends."

Emily said: "You don't have to grieve for your son yet. He is not dead. The HIV won't kill him for a long time. The drugs might."

I remembered that two years ago Emily had told me the same thing. Her simple words had enabled me to enjoy David's company and retake control of my life.

Emily and Alice, both of whom had drug-addicted children, comforted Lucy. "It took years for my son Mitchell to kick drugs." Emily said. "It happened only after everybody stopped enabling him. He hit rock bottom. He came around, and now he is OK, except for AIDS. But AIDS is easier to handle then drug dependence. It is a real disease and you don't have any choices. Unlike drugs, AIDS allows you to help your child, and be sad."

Alice added: "My daughter too quit only when she hit rock bottom. For years I paid her rent and bought her food, just so she would not sell her body. Finally I decided 'no more'. I took my granddaughter to my house and let my daughter manage on her own. It was very hard for me, but eventually she came around. She is healthy now and our relationship is not great, but OK. Unfortunately she became terribly jealous of Gilbert. Since he developed full-blown AIDS three years ago, he is the focus all my energies."We had all understood what she said. AIDS can stress a mother's relationship with her other children.

A few weeks later Lucy told us that Philip was out of jail. "The first day he slept at his brother's house, the next at his aunt's. Now he is back on the street. "I can't understand myself," she continued as if she were talking to herself. "Philip has disappointed me so often that I numb myself and stop caring. I put up a wall and feel nothing."

"I know what it feels like." Priscilla told her." I went through all that with Cathleen. You have already said everything there is to say. You've already pleaded about rehab, you've already threatened, coaxed, and cajoled. None of that worked. You simply have to 'turn yourself off'. It may not be nice, but that's what it comes down to. Think of it as if you were walking barefoot on concrete. If you keep walking, your feet form calluses. With drugs, your mind develops calluses."

"Sometimes when you do nothing you do something," Susan Katz said. "Not enabling him is doing something, even if it doesn't feel like it."

"Yes, I am learning to live for the moment," Lucy added. "I have times when my obsession and craziness go away…like when I sit here with you ladies, or when I make love to my boyfriend. I guess that's what life is all about now.

"But sometimes I just can't shut it out," Lucy said. "I get so mad and angry, I don't know what to do. Last week I really lost my temper. I was waitressing on Valentine's Day and the restaurant was packed. I gave my drink order to the bartender. When I put my tray on the bar, that schmuck said: 'Be careful, watch my birthday cake.'

"It was a piece of real gooey cheesecake, covered with whipped cream and raspberry sauce. I looked the guy straight in the face, picked up the cake and threw it at him. It felt so good, even though I had to jump through hoops all evening to get my work done."

Christmas, the traditional season for merriment, had come around. The group had its annual feast that reflected our diversified ethnic backgrounds. There was roasted pork from Uruguay, collard greens from the Deep South, Viennese cakes, French paté, rum-soaked fruitcake from Jamaica, latkes and blintzes. We had eaten as much as we could, taking the leftovers to Bailey House, a nearby AIDS residence.

As usual, buying gifts for David had alleviated my anxiety. I had sent eight presents, one for each night of Chanukah. He called, ecstatic. My grandchildren gave me an excuse to go back to F.A.O. Schwarz. How toys had changed since my children were small. I missed my Mom, whose favorite holiday Christmas had been. I was glad when the annual madness was over and I no longer felt duty-bound to say that I had had a great holiday.

◆   ◆   ◆

The Mothers' Group knew that Patrick had died shortly after Christmas. Maggie, his mother, was to come early in January to tell us how it had been. I dreaded the meeting, anticipating the day that I too might have to tell the group how it ended for David and me. Maggie had been with the group for almost three years. She was both traditional and unconventional, shy and daring. She was so gentle that I could not imagine her speaking with a raised voice.

Patrick had been a well-known jazz musician and composer. He had contracted AIDS sometimes at the beginning of the epidemic and now his health was failing. His illness had been very protracted.

"Patrick died last Wednesday," Maggie told us. "He was just tired of being sick. During the last months there had been one little thing after another and he was really going downhill."

We had always envied the Jessups' fun-filled Christmas. As usual they had gone caroling on Charles Street in Greenwich Village, lit their tree, and opened their presents.

Then they had all gone to their country house in Connecticut. "Patrick was too sick to be up," Maggie said, and he stayed in his room surrounded by his keyboards. Several of his very good friends came to see him and made him laugh.

"By Tuesday night, Patrick had trouble breathing. My husband and I stayed with him. He was not in pain, but we felt that he was going. Towards morning we went to bed to take a nap. Our daughter woke us, Patrick called out 'Mom,' went into respiratory failure, and was gone. "He had told us that he wanted to be buried in Connecticut. We called the funeral home, but since it was New Year's Day it took them some time to come. So Patrick was with us all day long and we could say goodbye.

"I pulled up the blankets over his shoulders so as to keep him warm. We all went in his room from time to time. I patted his cheek. It felt good to touch him, but it was no longer Patrick. His spirit had gone elsewhere.

"Something peculiar happened when the men from the funeral home finally wheeled out Patrick's body. We heard a loud bang, as if something had fallen. I ran upstairs to investigate, and a large old mirror had dropped off the wall and on to the dresser below it, but it had not broken. It was as if it were a sign from Patrick and he was saying goodbye."

"We buried Patrick in the little cemetery by the church I pass when I go shopping. It is a lively place where kids like to play and ride their bikes. Patrick would have liked that."

We were quiet after Maggie finished speaking. Finally Susan Katz said: "It is really very important to say goodbye. I believe that one can feel the spirit leave the body.

"My brother's death was not peaceful," Susan recalled. "My parents had not signed a DNR [Do Not Resuscitate]order. When Dan went into respiratory failure, the hospital personnel tried to resuscitate him. It is terrifying to watch such 'coding.' It looks as if the patient is physically abused and violated."

For Susan, ten years had not erased the horror.

"When the coding was over," Susan continued, "and Dan was gone, I asked the nurse to get all the medical equipment out of the room. Then we went in one by one to say goodbye.

"The next day we had services for Dan in a little old synagogue on the Lower East Side. The night following the services the synagogue burned to the ground.

"Neither my father nor I could sleep that night. We both got up and met in the kitchen. Two gas jets were burning. I know that my brother had not been ready to go, and his spirit was restless."

We were silent. There was so much pain and so much to do. We knew that we needed one another. We understood what each of us was going through. We could never again be the women we had once been. We were no better or worse, we simply were different. The concern of many old friends, even the sympathetic ones, simply didn't fit anymore.

After the formal portion of the meeting was over, we usually were exhausted from all the shared heartache. To regain some balance we went to Daisy's, a coffee shop on Seventh Avenue around the corner from Eleventh Street. The waiters and waitresses knew us and were always extra nice, even though some of us had only a cup of coffee.

It so happened that at Daisy's we shared our space with a group of transvestites and transsexuals with whom we had established a rapport. By now we know some of the "girls'" problems. They said they wished that their mothers were as understanding of them as we were of our children. "Your sons are lucky," one of them said.

I looked at my oddly assorted friends from the Mothers' Group and at these colorful creatures with their ropes of pearls, long peroxided hair, and garish make-up. "What was I doing here?" I wondered.

"Why did AIDS descend upon the world during the few years that I was here?" I mused. "Why was I no longer in my well-ordered childhood home in Hanover? I knew that the safety I felt then was illusory. If my family had stayed, the Nazis would have beaten down our front door and sent us to a gas chamber. Was any place safe? Is there any happiness left for me after AIDS?"

After Daisy's I boarded the subway. The familiar ride always cleared my mind. "David is different," the wheels sang, "it will be OK." Indeed, within a few weeks my apartment on Sanchez Street would be available. I would look at my healthy son and leave the New York winter behind.

I flew to San Francisco on a Friday. Two days later, on February 19th, about 15 of David's friends came to my loft to celebrate his birthday. We drank champagne and David was happy with his loot. What a big kid he was, my 37-year-old son!

A few days after David's 37th birthday party, his dark mood surfaced. "I've always had this thing with numbers," he told me. Aware of his fetish, I had adopted some of his "numbers." Like David, I warmed my coffee in the microwave for 2'19" (his birthday)—or 2'56" (his birth year.) "Well," David continued, "the other day I subtracted 19 from 56 and came up with 37, my present age!! Is this my last birthday?"

He had jotted down some of these thoughts in his diary: February 20, 1993: "I woke up on the morning after my 37th birthday and felt restless. I have to stop just marking time. There is so much I want to do and no matter how much time I have left in this life I better start doing it: Acting classes/writing a book/script/journal/tons of letters/reading a ton of books."

On March 27, David left for South America. He had accumulated enough Uninited airline milage for a free ticket, and the trip was going to cost him very little. He was traveling with Keith Potter and Keith's lover, Frank. The main purpose of the trip was to meet up with Jeff White, one of the Seven Sisters, who was working for the Peace Corps in Bogota, Columbia.

9

MOUNT ZION

"Rio," David wrote in his diary on March 28, 1993, *"is very relaxed, warm and humid. So far, aside from some begging, haven't experienced how dangerous people were saying it is."*

David had started his vacation with his usual energy: *"After getting into room, went to gay beach at Panema, walked, swam, ate (fish, risotto with chicken) napped, ate again, (steak and fries), then danced at Le Boy."*

After a few days Keith, Frank and David flew to Buenos Aires, where they met up with Jeff White, who was *"looking great, especially considering that he had been on a bus for 1 1/2 days."*

David ended up by disliking Buenos Aires heartily, perhaps because by then he was not feeling well. According to his diary he was *just a little grumpy and tired,"* his feet ached, and when dinner came he was not that hungry and gave away most of his food.

One week into the trip David called us in New York. He said that he was short of breath, that breathing deeply hurt, and that he had night sweats.

My chest also tightened. Here was another step along that treacherous path. Anyone familiar with AIDS might suspect that David was coming down with pneumonia.

David's next phone call, on April 7th, was from San Francisco. He had shortened his trip by a few days to seek medical care. A week later he retold the events in a letter to Jeff White:

Dear Jeff,

Well, its been exactly one week since we parted company—I figure I'll try to write to you sooner rather than later, especially since there is a lot to tell Unfortunately, my worst fears were realized and I have PCP (pneumocystis pneumonia).

It was very smart of me to leave early—I'm sure that every day makes a difference.

They say it's a mild case and I'm not being treated in a hospital, but it is still pretty awful and demoralizing.

The trip back was hellish, it appeared to be touch and go whether I would get on the Buenos Aires—Miami flight (it was totally full). Finally I did, but then there were more problems with the way they loaded the luggage, and we had to return to the gate, etc, etc. We got to Miami after 6 AM, and I rushed through the airport with my bags, sweating and coughing, and basically I almost killed myself.

Then I made the mistake of telling the stewardess about my condition and then they tried to harass me into getting off the plane. It was horrible, and I will complain. (The stewardess finally called her supervisor, who was gay, and who let David take the trip.)

Kathy (Dickie) met me at the gate, which was great. Crystal (Robert Driscoll) had made a doctor's appointment. I had an x-ray, and the next day (Thursday) they called me and told me it was abnormal—that led to more tests and a diagnosis on Friday. Luckily there's a new treatment (an oral antibiotic called Mepron) which hopefully I can tolerate and will work.

I guess I'm sort of stunned right now. I'm just trying to focus on getting over this and then move on with my life.

My mother flew out Sunday night—thank God—I really don't know what I would do without her here—you really need someone dedicated to you to help.

Now regarding the mail—my birthday card (very cute) was waiting for me when I got back.

Friday 4/16/93

...I am doing better. They also prescribed prednisone (steroids) on Wednesday, which seems to have helped a lot with the coughing spasms & fevers. I'm tapering them off. I'll be feeling better daily now.

What nightmare, though! It's really hard to keep negative thoughts (which I hate) out.

Back to the mail and your shopping list...

As David had written in his letter to Jeff, Dr. Gilmore, one of Dr. Conant's assistants, had diagnosed PCP, the disease that had felled so many AIDS patients at the beginning of the epidemic. Now, in 1993, 97 percent of all AIDS patients recovered from their first episode of PCP. Fortunately, David had a mild case, and there was no need for hospitalization. Gilmore prescribed Mepron, a new oral antibiotic. Nevertheless, both the doctor and my son were shocked by David's immune profile: 20 T cells and very few helper cells!

I had a hard time being matter-of-fact when David called us in New York with this latest news. It was as if the second shoe I had expected for all these years had dropped. I hoped that I sounded cool, calm and reassuring on the phone. Fortunately, David did not sound that sick. I delayed flying out to California for a few days because of Adam Balzano.

◆　　　◆　　　◆

Two months after their Hawaii trip, Rhea had once more taken Adam to the hospital. Upon admission he had said, "Mom, I think I won't get out of the hospital this time."

"Adam, you don't know," Rhea had answered. "I am not ready to let go."

"Mom," Adam replied, "I am not ready to let go either, but sometimes one does not have a choice."

He died on March 15th, as he had wanted, in total control of his life. Rhea scheduled a memorial for the week that David had returned so precipitously from South America, and I wanted to be with my friend.

◆　　　◆　　　◆

The day after the event, Ernest took me to Newark airport well ahead of time. We were frightened for our son and held hands. Then I was facing the immediate future alone.

I had savored the many years that David had been symptom-free, trying to prepare myself for the day that he might become ill. Yet in no way was I ready to confront overt disease. I still could not say: "My son has AIDS."

The magic of soaring into the sky had never quite left me. I loved being in the air, safe from intrusions. During many trips out to California I had joyfully anticipated my visits with my son. Now I was panicky. How would David be when I got there? I knew that I could not collapse, and had to be cheerful, confident and competent.

David met me at the airport. He was tense, but sported a tan and looked as handsome as ever. Back at the apartment, Liza greeted me in her nonchalant way.

David handed me the present he had brought for me from South America—a leather frame for my mother's picture. Then Robert Driscoll picked him up for an evening out.

It was almost as if David had waited for my arrival to get really ill. He coughed more, vomited and breathed very poorly. At times he gasped for air, and the oxygen shortage caused anxiety attacks. He moaned and kept repeating, "Mommy, Mommy, help; Mommy, Mommy, help." The incantation disturbed me greatly, since I was powerless in the face of this dreadful disease. I asked David to stop imploring me. He said that my name was sort of a mantra for him, which he used even when I was not there.

In spite of his being so sick, I was happy to be with David. I felt privileged that he let me take care of him. I thought that I would resent being a "nurse," but to my surprise, did not mind.

Long ago I had trained myself to postpone fear until a crisis had resolved itself. Now my calm somewhat diffused David's hysteria.

I knew how scared my poor son was. He had been infected with the HIV virus in 1983 and now, a decade later, there still was no effective treatment. Neither David, nor his doctors, nor I, however, believed that this pneumonia was going to do him in. We feared, however, that it was the beginning of the long downward spiral characteristic of AIDS.

Instead of verbalizing our dread, David and I talked, as we always did, of nothing and everything—the trips we had taken—the ones we were going to take. It was just a year ago that we had rented a condominium on Kauai. We conjured up our two lanais, the birds that shared our breakfast, the whales that passed in the nearby ocean, the overflowing washing machine, our favorite among the "hidden" beaches to which we carted gourmet lunches, complete with cocktails. We promised ourselves to return to Kauai as soon as we could.

We cheered ourselves up recalling other funny events that had occurred as we wined and dined over the years: a horribly overpriced cognac here, a maître-d' so voluble that our food grew cold, the owner of a B & B who masterfully conned us out of breakfast. We were so attuned to one another that there was seldom a cross word. I made a supreme effort to keep the house as neat as David liked it to be, and he was grateful.

David's nights were worse than his days. His fever spiked. He coughed and vomited. When I lay on my makeshift bed in the living room, I listened to him as I used to when he was an infant. I was up whenever I felt he needed me. We slept very little, and once I was so tired that I crept into his bed. I told David of Carmen, one of the mothers of my group, who woke up one night because her son's overtired night nurse slipped into her bed. We laughed.

On Tuesday after I arrived we went to see Mark Illeman, David's trusted physician assistant. Mark and David hugged. My son cried. "When I am over this, I want to reexamine my whole treatment scheme," David said. Mark prescribed some cough medication and Naprosyn, a more effective anti-pyretic than aspirin. I asked whether Mepron was really effective against PCP and Mark assured me that Conant's office was part of the official clinical trial of that new drug. David showed Mark a tiny red sore on the sole of his foot. "No," Mark said, "it is definitely not KS."

Mark tested David's blood oxygenation. It was lower than it had been the previous Friday. Nobody worried, attributing the poor results to a difference in the measuring technique. In retrospect, this should have been a major cause for alarm.

The next day, Wednesday, we saw Gilmore. I liked this young, conscientious physician. I was impressed by his care and concern. He was surprised that I had come out to San Francisco to be there for David. Mothers supporting their ailing sons still seemed to be a rarity. Gilmore added cortisone (Prednisone). David showed Gilmore the little red spot on his foot. Gilmore also did not believe it was it was KS.

Time took on an air of unreality. It was both long and short. The world outside David's apartment shrank, and inconsequential events assumed gigantic proportions. And yet, in spite of impending doom, life maintained its typical rhythm of small pleasures and miseries.

David and I felt an immense tenderness for each other, sensing that life as we knew it was about to change. Sometimes I invited friends for dinner, but their company was almost too taxing. One evening, as we played solitaire on my computer, David told me that he liked best spending the evening alone with me. I hoped that I would never forget the surge of love and loss I experienced. Nobody ever would feel that way about me again.

By the end of the week David seemed to improve, but not fast enough. The guy who covered for the doctor that weekend prescribed some more cough medicine and told us to be patient.

Friends came to visit, including Dave Nelson—who had already had several AIDS-related opportunistic infections—and his HIV-negative partner, Robert Wagner. The two just had fulfilled one of their dreams: buying their own home. They discussed furniture, paint and wallpaper. What guts it must take to plan for an ordinary life when death is staring you in the face!

For years, Frank Hawkins and David had had an on-again-off-again friendship. Now Frank came over to make peace. Frank's T-cells had dropped below one hundred. Still, he kept up his swimming, and even qualified for several competitive events. Two years hence, New York was to host the Gay Olympics, and Frank planned to come and stay with us then. How could he plan that far ahead? I wondered.

On Wednesday, April 21, we went back to see Gilmore, who declared that David "moves air around his lungs more easily than last week." Gilmore assured us that David was getting better. When I asked whether it was OK for me to leave the coming weekend, Gilmore answered, "no problem." He told David to take it easy and not to return to work too soon. He ordered a follow-up x-ray for May 11—five weeks after the original one. He also filled out Workman's Compensation forms for AT & T, speculating that David would be out until the middle of May. David glanced at the diagnosis Gilmore had scribbled on the form: It had changed from HIV to AIDS. "I knew it," David said with despair and rage.

Gilmore was leaving for Washington to celebrate Gay Pride Day and march down the Mall with one million others. As in 1979 and 1989, David too had hoped to be there marching together with Stewart Mittler, his friend from college.

Since this was a Wednesday, there was a theater matinee. We got tickets for Dinner at Eight, one of David's favorites. He recalled previous productions and the actors in the movie version, and started to recite the play's dialogue. David had a hard time walking up the stairs of the theater. Never mind; for a few hours we happily forgot about our troubles.

◆   ◆   ◆

My gut feeling was that we had not yet seen the end of this pneumonia. David seemed to get weaker instead of better. On Thursday night he had a high fever. On Friday he was too wiped out to get out of bed.

Alice Fallon, from my Mothers' Group, was in San Francisco to bid farewell to her son Gilbert. For years, Alice and I had felt close because of our common San Francisco connection. Gilbert, a Brother of the Franciscan order, lived around the corner from David. I had sneaked out several times to be with Alice, but had not told David that Gilbert was dying. I knew that my son did not want to deal with "negative thoughts."

That Saturday afternoon I had to tell him that I would attend Gilbert's memorial. The celebratory Mass, held in a sun-drenched chapel, was in sharp contrast with the sadness everyone felt. Even though Gilbert had violated the order's vow of chastity, his superior raged against the disease that was killing some of the world's best citizens. Alice wore the elegant white dress her son had given the previous Christmas.

Before returning to my own heartache, I stopped at a local Safeway, where Calistoga Spring Water was on sale. Under the circumstances, the price of the water was trivial, yet I struggled with the weight of a dozen quart bottles How could I let such a trivial saving intrude on my collapsing universe?

While I was out, David and Robert Driscoll had gone to the park across the street. The small expedition had exhausted David totally.

On Sunday, David was even worse. He could barely shower, and panted when he spoke. I called Rob Saper, Judy's friend and a smart family practitioner. He was surprised that "the guys" working for Conant did not follow David's pulmonary function more closely." Sam Sklar, my New Jersey doctor friend, felt the same when I consulted him.

At 3 PM I insisted that we go to the emergency room at Mount Zion Hospital. Unfortunately, I had been correct. David's pneumonia was not improving; his blood oxygen level was extremely low.

"You know that we are going to admit you to the hospital," the resident told David, who was already comfortably stretched out on a cot. Nurses had provided him with an oxygen mask, threaded a thin plastic cannula through his nose and had wheeled him to the fifth floor. With the extra oxygen, David felt better. It was hard for us to grasp the reality of the situation.

Since Gilmore was in Washington, Dr. Marge Poscher assumed David's medical care. With her boyish haircut, metal-rimmed glasses and tie, she was most attractive, a real "dyke" doctor, as David described her affectionately on the phone to his friend Andrea Lepcio. In time David and I got to like Poscher very much.

Poscher started David on IV pentamadine and a high dosage of corticosteroids—2400 mg/day. We were shocked and hopeful. That evening I returned alone to David's apartment. I walked Liza, took a sleeping pill, and slept rather well. I couldn't afford to think.

Monday: I arrived early at the hospital. "I missed you," David said. My mind soaked up every word as if it knew it would treasure these minute details in the years to come. Our spirits were high. The IV pentamadine would do the trick. Flowers kept arriving. David's friends came to visit en masse. Poscher was confident.

All hospitals are depressing, though this one was better than most. The male and female nurses in the small, 15-bed AIDS unit were nice, even if not always smart. The food was good. Visiting hours were unlimited.

Room 543—our home—was quite comfortable. It was large enough to accommodate a television, a VCR and an entire flower shop. A former AIDS patient had donated a floor-wide audio system, and each room had a fancy CD player and earphones. Every night before leaving, I selected some music for David to listen to during the night.

My poor son continued to be brave and scared. Despite his general debilitation he also was his usual energetic self, enjoying the general bustle. It was hard to cope with the steady flow of visitors, the constantly ringing phone, and the therapy appointments David set up with Margie. He needed more oxygen when he talked, and the long conversations tired him.

I started to screen David's calls. In sign language I asked whether he wanted to talk himself or have me handle it. I made mental notes of the snatches of conversations I overheard when he took the phone:

"The first two days [after I got to the hospital] I was in absolute shock. I was such a good patient—I did everything I could. They just fucked up. Then the next two days I was angry and did not know where to put my anger. Now I can start to deal with it."

Another conversation: "You should see my room, so full of flowers." Sick as he was, he derived much pleasure from his nieces describing them as: "Naomi, the little tomboy and Ana, the little Miss Muffet, who wants to get her ears 'pissed'. "Naomi," he reported, "still tries to get the boys to play with her."

Nobody worried much about David's illness when he was at home, but now everybody was upset. At Seventeenth Street too the phone was ringing constantly in the morning before I got to the hospital, during the day, and in the evening after I got home: Patt Argiro, Debra Shine, my sister, Andrea, Susan Katz, Rhea, Judy Powsner, Stewart, Joseph, Jim, Anne, Judy, Ernest….

Tons of friends appeared at the hospital: Dave Nelson, Frank Hawkins, Gary Kukus, people from AT&T, Alan, Rick, David's Halloween crowd, his school friends….

San Francisco's AIDS network swung into action. Two lawyers appeared. They wanted to help David make a will. David was business-like and upset. After a short while I threw the lawyers out. There was a social worker, an art therapist, and an organization ready to deliver meals after David got home.

I was in the hospital from early in the morning to late at night. I didn't want to be elsewhere. I was at peace being with David. I tried to keep him quiet and relaxed. To save his breath we started writing to each other on a yellow pad of paper.

Poscher kept adding more antibiotics. David's anxiety level increased. He had the nurses check his oxygenation level every few hours. When the numbers were up, he rejoiced, when they were down he was dejected. He developed hemorrhoids and had trouble moving his bowels.

Margie, his therapist, brought him a Teddy bear and made him a relaxation tape. "Think about Provincetown, Wellfleet, or Hawaii," we told him. He enjoyed listening to stories of long ago, and I racked my brain to come up with new ones. I was so sad, but sometimes when my voice became veiled with tears, David told me sternly: "Mother, don't cry."

Rarely David shifted to another level of consciousness. "Just in case...Ana gets Cher, Naomi gets Bette Mitler, and Sean gets Zero Mostel." I had bought David his first Hirschfeld lithograph when he had graduated from high school, and acquiring others had been our common project ever since. He reminded me that he wanted to leave a little bit of money to many different people, hoping that they would spend it thinking of him. He wanted to draw up a list of the intended recipients. I vetoed the plan. "Why,"?" he asked. "It might be fun."

I managed to ask him whether he wanted to be cremated and "snuggle in" with his grandmother at Ferncliffe cemetery. He asked where I would be. "With you," I told him. I couldn't believe that this was really happening.

When David was in such a down mood he looked at all the flowers and the cards and quoted John, an old date, now long dead: "The first time you go to the hospital everybody gets very upset and sends you flowers and cards...by the fifth time everybody is bored with you...."

Fortunately we were not yet there. By Monday of the second week Conant finally appeared. David was happy to see him, and Conant cheered him up. "This is not the time to be scared," Conant said. "If you become scared, you'll die." When David pointed out that Gilmore and Illeman should have taken his condition more seriously in the beginning, Conant promised to discuss the matter later. "Not now," Conant kept insisting.

During the next few days Conant was very attentive, and called David from the airport and from Washington, where he was helping Clinton to pick an AIDS tsar.

The days dragged on. David was not really getting better. He seemed to need more oxygen. Nobody bothered giving him a sponge bath, and on Monday he ventured into the shower tethered to a movable oxygen tank. In spite of the oxygen he nearly collapsed. Initially David had still eaten with his usual relish, but as the days passed and he required additional oxygen, eating became more difficult.

Poscher added Clindamycin, a nasty antibiotic which upset David's stomach. He also strained at stool and became exhausted when he went to the bathroom. At my urging, the nurses produced a commode.

The random notes on the big yellow pad were getting more desperate and frustrated:

"I have to calm down right now."

"I am glad you are here. I need to relax. I can't deal with too many doctors, you need to help."

"They came in the middle of the night to give me yet another respiratory treatment."

"Poscher still added another antibiotic."

Some notes were typically David: A daily list of what to tell the doctor; a detailed chronicle of what had happened during the night while I was gone, musings about what music to load onto the CD player, who was in which movie, how much I had to pay the maid. Exhortations about remaining optimistic: "We shouldn't get excited about the [chest] x-ray whatever it says." I am surprised how often my son reassured me of his love for me.

There was one very hopeful note: "Maybe we should save this pad as a record of our stay in the hospital."

David hated being ill. "I never want to be that sick again," he told me. "Right," I said out loud, but inwardly, having watched the sons of my friends suffer for years, I feared that I knew what was in store for him.

We got the hang of the hospital and of the staff. Many of the nurses were excellent, a few were middling. Sandra, a tall blonde, who David assumed was a transsexual, amused us. At the nurses' station I overheard somebody referring to her as "Nurse Ratchet" from *One Flew Over the Cuckoo's Nest*. I told David and we laughed.

I loved the quiet evenings when the bustle of the hospital had died down. We watched television and videotapes of favorite old movies.

David seemed to be deteriorating. On Wednesday he had almost collapsed while sitting on the commode. The nurses had been ready to send out an alert. Fortunately Gilmore, who happened to be on the hospital floor, canceled the order. Gilmore had summoned a respiratory therapist who provided David with a fancier oxygen mask and aggressive therapy.

Thursday Poscher had told me that David had very low oxygen reserves and that she was trying her best to keep him breathing on his own "until that pneumonia turns around." The she asked me to try to keep him quiet. I had succeeded in stemming the flow of visitors, but some had slipped through. It did not seem to matter. David's spirit was undaunted. When there were no visitors he had long talks with the hospital orderlies.

Ernest and Judy debated about who would fly out first to visit us. It was decided that Judy would come on Friday, May 7, and stay for the weekend. I don't know who was more relieved to see her walk in, David or me. I loved being with both of my children. "Perhaps this is the last time you'll have them both," a little voice squeaked in my head. I squelched the thought.

On his yellow pad David wrote to Judy: "Its so good to have you here, also for Mommy. It's been a big strain." Then he added: "In many! (underlined three times) years the kids will get lots of life insurance money from AT & T."

I looked at Judy and David. Even after almost forty years, I found it miraculous that they had emerged from my loins. Judy massaged David's back, propped him up comfortably and was very loving. I left them alone.

Frank Hawkins took me for a walk on the Marine Headlands. We ended up at the Cliff House, a restaurant gift shop sitting on a cliff promontory overlooking San Francisco Bay. We looked at the churning sea and discussed how we would try to clamber out, if per chance we fell into the swirling waters. We were completely engrossed in our game, and for ten minutes forgot the real abyss that was engulfing David, Frank and me.

Sunday morning I arrived at the hospital at about nine. Judy came a bit later. David greeted us with a big smile. During the night he had again needed an extra visit by the respiratory specialist. Early that afternoon Judy shoed me out of the room. I was very reluctant to go, but also wanted my children to have time by themselves.

I didn't know what to do with myself. I went home and walked Liza. I drove downtown to go swimming. Before I got there I turned around. Finally I wound up in the Castro movie theater, watching Katherine Hepburn, Jimmy Stewart and Cary Grant in "The Philadelphia Story," even becoming absorbed in the plot. When it was over I rushed to Mount Zion. David was exhausted. Twenty minutes after I got there he had a coughing fit. His eyes turned upward; he was in respiratory failure. The nurse sounded the alarm. Suddenly the room was filled with blue-clad bodies. They worked on David and told Judy and me to leave the room. The two of us stood outside helplessly. We watched the blue-clad army wheel David out of his room, down to the intensive care unit (ICU).

Ruth, Rob and Shoshana Saper, who had planned to visit, appeared. All of us were miserable and speechless. I called Ernest in New York. "We lost him," was all I could say.

◆   ◆   ◆

David's bed was in a rather spacious plexiglass-enclosed cubicle at the very end of the ICU. He was intubated, but still looked good. He still smiled, and an attendant dubbed him Smiley. He could not talk. Sometimes they tied his hands to prevent him from accidentally pulling out the tube attached to the respirator.

Though there was nothing for me to do, I spent all my day at the hospital. If I had not been so tired I would have spent the night, too. Ernest arrived on Monday. When David saw him he smiled. He motioned for his big yellow writing pad, and on it scribbled the name of a restaurant we should go to.

The Loebl family took over the waiting room of the ICU. It was comfortably furnished with big blue couches, armchairs and a huge television set. Judy had stayed until Wednesday, before returning to New York. By then Andrea, David's trusted "girlfriend," and her lover, Lynn, had arrived. Like Ernest and me, they camped out in the waiting room of the ICU. David recognized Andrea, and wrote in big letters, "I won't die."

Judy Powsner, his friend from Brandeis, flew in from Boston. David's San Francisco friends: Robert Driscoll, Robert Wagner, Frank Hawkins, Alan Crouch, his cousin Jim Lewinson, Cindy and many more checked in regularly, but most were not allowed into the ICU proper. At first I was a little put out by all these people, but then I appreciated their support and the tremendous love David had inspired in all of us. One surprise visitor was Jeff Price, David's long lost lover. Jeff was terribly distraught. How I wished David would know.

David had a harder and harder time communicating. He was thirsty, but all we could give him was ice-chips. When we didn't understand what he wanted, David got very excited and his oxygen requirements increased. Andrea and Lynn made him a little book with statements he could point to, but the distance between David and us grew.

Poscher finally concluded that the pentamadine had not worked. She managed to get a new, experimental medication from the NIH—trimethotrexate—an anti-folate drug closely related to cancer agents. I wondered why it had taken her that long to try this drug.

David developed a bacterial pneumonia on top of his *pneumocystis*. He had a fever. He was heavily sedated: valium, morphine and Pavulon—a paralyzing drug that was supposed to reduce the discomfort of the breathing tube.

The nursing staff in the ICU was great. They all seemed to like David, and were truly impressed by the support his family gave him. They even worried about me. Once when I was sobbing while talking on the pay phone in the hall, a nurse rushed over with a box of Kleenex. A resident brought a pillow when he saw me stretched out on a couch in the waiting room. "See," he said, "we have all those beds here. We don't want you in one of them. Take care of yourself, eat, sleep."

I did not want to sleep. All I wanted was to sit by David's bed. His feet were uncovered, unencumbered by high-tech machinery. I kept looking at them. The little red mark that had worried him so much was still there. The regular sound of the respirator was soothing. I made believe that David was little, or that we were on Kauai or at home. I told David that I was there. I couldn't quite tell him anymore that he would make it.

We were starting our second week in the ICU. Poscher was hopeful. David's fever had abated. The bacterial pneumonia was gone, as was the *pneumocystis*. David, however, could no longer breathe on his own or even tolerate a lowering of the oxygen level.

The doctors were baffled. They had expected David to get better or worse, not to stabilize on the respirator. Poscher feared that David had developed Adult Respiratory Failure Syndrome—a fancy way of saying that his lungs were shot. The doctor hinted that we might have to turn off the respirator. This was shit on top of shit. I thought of my friend Blanche Mednick, who after seven weeks had had to take the responsibility of turning off Brian's respirator.

We were not quite ready to make this decision. We asked Rob Saper to sit in on a conference with Poscher. We called Ian Shine, our British physician friend now living in New York. Ian understood what we were going through. A few months earlier his daughter Cathy had suffered from a near-fatal asthma attack, and eventually the Shines too had to give permission to turn off the respirator.

Ian unearthed a Yale doctor specializing in adult respiratory distress syndrome. The Yale man advised us to wait. Ian offered to fly to San Francisco and talk to Poscher. We settled for a telephone conference. Ian listened to Poscher, and agreed with her that David's condition was hopeless.

I had called my New York internist, Kenneth Praeger, who happened to be a lung specialist. He too had said that we should wait another week. We deferred the decision to turn off the respirator until Monday.

The long countdown began. I knew that we would have to turn off the respirator on Monday. David was not getting any better and every few hours or so his blood pressure shot up and his pulse raced. Then the staff calmed him down with more sedatives. As I sat by his bed, watching the monitor gyrate wildly, I heard myself say: "Kick it boy, kick it."

Judy had flown out again, this time bringing two-year old Sean. I had not realized how much I needed her. Sean added variety to our long vigil in the ICU. We took turns watching him. He was a very good boy.

I'll never forget that interminable weekend. How could I acquiesce in turning off the respirator? How could I take a chance of not turning it off? Poscher said that David might not remain as comfortable as he seemed to be now. How did we know that David was not suffering? I felt totally helpless and cried whenever I was by myself.

Ernest had a different attitude. He talked to everybody on the staff, trying to find out whether there was any hope for David to recover. At one point he even found some residents who told him that they would "wake David up" so that he could talk to us.

Monday came around. I had dressed carefully, as I knew David would have liked me to. When I got to the hospital, Robert Driscoll was already there. The nurse untied David's hands and told us to prevent him from pulling out his respiratory tube. "He is very weak, so it won't be difficult to restrain him." she said. Indeed, when David raised the hand, whose feel I loved so much, it was enough for me to hold it lightly. I talked to Robert. David heard us, opened his eyes and bestowed his warm, luminous smile on us. We talked to him, and soon he drifted off.

Poscher came. She was visibly shaken and requested one more carbon dioxide level. It came back higher (worse) than before. Even all the oxygen could no longer cleanse David's blood. Poscher ordered the withdrawal of life support. The nurses gave David some more morphine. Slowly his blood oxygenation dropped from 95 to 90 to 80…. Life ebbed out of my son. We were all there: Ernest, Judy, me and even Sean.

I tried hard not to be corny. Still, I remembered the day 37 year ago when he was born, and the traditional Jewish prayer: "God gives and God takes and His name be praised."

10

GRIEF

"We are starting our descent to San Francisco," the pilot announced. "We should be at the gate in 30 minutes." My heart skipped a beat. I had flown to California so often during the last decade, certain of the love awaiting me. Now that was gone.

The flight had been less painful than expected. I had sat next to an attractive reporter from the Oakland Tribune. He was attentive, and had regaled me with some of his journalistic exploits. Our conversation had the intimacy of strangers whose lives touched for a brief moment. Our small talk kept me from disintegrating.

I had not asked any of David's friends to meet me at the airport. I dislike people witnessing my raw grief, and I hurt too much to smile. So I took the Super-shuttle, my son's chatter reverberating in my head:

"You are back home," he used to say. "How does it feel? See Candlestick Park? The Giants threaten to move because the wind impacts on the ball." Or: "I should have taken [highway] 280 this time of the day. Liza will be so happy to see you. I want to take you to brunch at that new place on Guerrero. The plants need haircuts. You have to iron some shirts...."

I unlocked the door of the apartment. Everything was as I had left it three weeks ago: The Hirschfeld lithographs lined the hall; the enormous philodendron, grown from a cutting smuggled into California from our first trip to Hawaii, was still green, the geraniums I had planted in the window box to cheer up the air shaft were flowering; the pictures and notices plastered on the refrigerator door were still there, and so was the freezer filled with the food I had cooked months ago. Yet everything was different: David was missing and Liza was back East with Stewart until we could take her.

The three weeks I had spent in New York had been awfully long and very short. Most often "I was" still with David on Seventeenth Street or in the hospital. I didn't want to let go. I was afraid to forget. I couldn't believe that he was gone.

My unconscious knew. For years, each time the phone rang I expected it to be David. Now I knew that it was not he.

My one consolation was that for David AIDS had been relatively benign. I remembered when he told me, in the hospital, that he never wanted to be that sick again. He kept his word to himself. Perhaps we do have some control over when we die. But I also remembered David telling me how much he loved life and how hard it was leaving it.

Back in New York I had talked to many of my friends, and had seen some, but was most comfortable when alone. I could respond to art and beauty. Once I had gone to the ballet, and cried non-stop as Balanchine's *Jewels* unfolded on the stage. I had visited Fort Tryon Park, and looked down at the Hudson as it bathed Manhattan. I used to go to that park often when the children were small. A lifetime earlier, I had gone there with a Turkish boyfriend. The mighty river reminded him of the Bosphorus in Istanbul. It was comforting to know that the river would be here long after I too was gone.

I wished for that time to be now. I felt aimless, but sensed that my job here on earth was not yet done. I wanted to keep David's memory alive. I wanted to be there for Ernest, Judy and her children. And yes, if I could, I wanted to pass on what I had learned to others. I envied those who believed in a hereafter. How much lighter my grief would be if I were convinced that I would see David again.

How did one grieve, anyway? Self-help books seemed trite. The memories of those who'd lost a lover, a brother, a child, a parent, were better. I read Paul Monnette's *Borrowed Time,* John Gunther's *Death Be Not Proud,* Barbara Ascher's *Landscape Without Gravity,* Isabel Allende's *Paula,* I watched *Shadow Land,* a love story that blossomed in the twilight between life and death.

Friends, old and new, sent cards and letters, some indifferent, some remarkably sensitive. People I never heard of shared my plight. Marge Poscher wrote, and Hiroko, the young Japanese woman who unquestioningly had sent David dextran sulfate at the beginning of the epidemic, sent flowers. Not everybody responded to my need. Some close friends were silent. Though they simply might have been unable to face my loss, or were afraid that my misfortune would "rub off," I was hurt. I realized that I was getting harder, more distant.

◆   ◆   ◆

The day after David died, we'd had a funeral service in San Francisco's Gay synagogue, where he had felt more at home than in any other temple. Rabbi Kahn, a gay man who with his partner had adopted a young son, had officiated. In his eulogy the rabbi had caught my son's spirit, his sense of fun and humor, his love for his family and friends, his anger and rage, his habit of never getting things done in time. The rabbi had concluded by reading the meditation on life by Rabbi Alvin Fine:

> Birth is a beginning and death a destination,
> But life is a journey,
> A going, a growing, from stage to stage
> From childhood to maturity, and youth to age,
> From innocence to awareness, and ignorance to knowing,
> From foolishness to discretion, and then perhaps to wisdom.
> From weakness to strength, or strength to weakness,
> And often back again,
> From health to sickness, and back to health again.
> From offense to forgiveness, from loneliness to love,
> From joy to gratitude, from pain to compassion,
> And grief to understanding, from fear to faith,
> From defeat, to defeat, to defeat,
> Until, looking backward or ahead,
> We see victory lies not at some high place along the way,
> But in having made the journey, stage by stage,
> A sacred pilgrimage.
> Birth is a beginning and death a destination.
> But life is a journey, a sacred pilgrimage,
> Made stage by stage, to life everlasting.

And "life everlasting" had been there at the service. In the total chaos that accompanies death, we had neglected to get a baby sitter for Sean. Impervious to the solemnity of the temple, David's two-year old nephew insisted on running around, vocalizing.

After the service I returned to New York. I had left my home precipitously when David had returned from South America, and after the six interminable weeks of David's illness I needed a break. I had come back to San Francisco to help Robert Driscoll organize "A Celebration of David Loebl's Life." That's what memorials are euphemistically called in the Time of AIDS.

Family and friends had flown in from all over the United States: Boston, New York City, New Jersey, Wisconsin, Cape Cod, Los Angeles—150 people in all. Susan Katz had been a welcome, unexpected guest. As master of ceremonies, Driscoll stated, "It was David's biggest party ever," and we knew that he would have loved it. There had been tons of food, music, dancing, gigantic props, flowers, rainbow-colored balloons, colorful table cloths, candles, photo albums, videotapes, slides. We had distributed photos of a happy David, red AIDS ribbons, and paper airplanes made by Ana and Naomi.

During two hours we had listened to those whose lives David had touched in so many different ways. I had spoken of the special relationship I had with my son, and of the loss whose depth I could not yet fathom.

Judy had spoken to her brother directly, recalling their intertwined lives:

"I remember the Saturday mornings before Mom and Dad got up, playing elaborate fantasy games in which our beds were boats and the floor was a dangerous ocean.

"And I remember how you saved the cherries from your cherry vanilla ice cream and ate them last; and how you teased me and drove me crazy; and how you always tried to make sure that things were fair in our family.

"David, I remember how you came out to me in a letter during your senior year in college. I remember feeling a sense of relief, feeling happy for you, feeling like you had found a missing piece in your life.

"And I remember going dancing together. Your enthusiasm and energy were contagious. I danced with you how I never danced with anyone else.

"I remember visiting you when I was pregnant with Ana and Naomi, and how proud and excited you were. And I remember, it was during that visit you found out you had only 180 T-cells. I cried the whole way home on the plane.

"And I remember Ana falling asleep on your shoulder when she was six weeks old and you came to meet your nieces for the first time. And I remember you trading riddles with Naomi last summer in Maine.

"And I remember how you made it back East every August to celebrate their birthday and to take the yearly Chanukah picture.

"And I remember coming to visit you last July with Sean, and how the two of you had breakfast together while I ran around Dolores Park.

"And I remember how scared you looked when I came to see you in the hospital.

"And I remember that you didn't want to die.

"David, I will always remember your sense of humor and your personal sense of history.

"I will always remember your loyalty, your desire to struggle things out, and your love.

"David, I will always talk to your spirit, carry you in my heart, and always, always will I remember you.

Robert Driscoll had spoken of their close friendship, and recalled his own annoyance, two weeks earlier, when David had failed to call and wish him a happy birthday.

My friend, Patt Argiro, had spoken of David, the toddler, "with a smile so wide that his big blue eyes had to squinch up to make room for it...and [of him] dancing, as soon as he could balance on two legs, with a decidedly theatrical flair."

Dancing had remained David's passion, akin to a religious experience. "In his love of dance David's soul," Robert Wagner had recalled, "his holiness was most clearly expressed...He was like a Dionysian reveler, celebrating at San Francisco's Box or at the I-Beam...."

Andrea could not face the reality of David's death. She sang of seeing David "sipping wine in a piazza. Sunning and feeling the soft warm breeze." Stewart Mittler had talked of their college years at Brandeis:

"Whenever David introduced me he would say: 'this is Stewart, one of my oldest friends.' He had called me to report that Shirley, [David's first dog] had died, and had said: 'now that Shirley is gone you and Judy Powsner are my oldest friends,' and I guess the title stuck.

"The idea that Shirley was his friend was one of the wonderful things about David. He had an innocence and exuberance about everything in life that was almost childlike, and this was combined paradoxically with a remarkable intellect and a sophisticated appreciation of art, music, theater and film."

In the beginning, David and Stewart's friendship had centered on films and dry martinis. They never tired of discussing movies, quoting their favorite lines, and "the martinis had been remarkable in improving the taste of the 'damn' dining hall food."

"David was a trusted confidant and friend," Stewart continued. "It always amazed me how good he was at giving advice. Whether the issues involved career, school, personal relationships, HIV, or just day-to-day living, David could sift through all the facts and consistently come up with the most logical solution...."

We also shared a sense of political commitment. This was instilled in us by our respective families originally, but it was nurtured...at Brandeis, a school where politics was very much part of everyday life...We took part in countless demonstrations together. Our first was a building takeover at Brandeis in 1975 to protest budget cuts that affected poor students. After that there were a multitude of gay pride marches in Boston and New York, then the two national marches on Washington in 1978 and 1987. I always loved marching with David, because he would get the entire crowd chanting along whatever the issue was, gay rights, AIDS funding, or economic fairness.

"Lastly I think the most important thing we shared was laughter, the basis of all truly great friendships. We could with one look, a gesture, or a phrase set each other off into spasms of laughter, often leaving onlookers completely bewildered, not quite getting it, wondering what was so funny. That's what made it so special...

"The last time I saw David was in Provincetown. The visit was very good. It involved many of our favorite things: a lobster dinner at Herring Cove, martinis and lots of laughter.... Michael Leak entertained us with his impersonations of semi-famous people. When he got to Eunice Kennedy Shriver, David and I were doubled up with laughter, tears streaming down our faces.

David and I...twenty years of shared laughter. I will miss the laughter more than I could possibly tell you here today, and I will cherish my memories until the day I die."

The celebration was over. My son had been loved and knew how to enjoy life. But why did we have to have a memorial? Why could it not have been a wedding, a birth, an anniversary?

My nephew, Jim Lewinson, was to be married in Carmel the week after the memorial, with David serving as his cousin's best man. With some misgivings, Ernest and I had decided to attend the wedding in spite of our loss.

Ernest and I spent the day before the wedding in Big Sur. We had dinner at the Ventana Inn. From its terrace we looked at the Pacific and the magnificent yellow hills bordering it. The juxtaposition of the wild and the civilized, of the sea, the land and the sky, was breathtaking. I felt close to the forces that shaped this earth.

My mind backtracked fifteen months. David and I were brunching on another terrace bordering the Pacific. This one was in Kauai, and the cliffs were those of the Napali coast. We were sipping champagne and feeling serene. "This is one of life's perfect moments," David had said, raising his glass. Several lizards darted in and out among the tables and chairs. One took a fancy to us and lingered. We snapped his picture.

Suddenly, as I sat on the terrace of the Ventana Inn, a lizard emerged from among the cracks in the rocks. It looked at me, blew up its fat cheeks and was in no hurry to go. Was it David's spirit telling me that he was here with me? I was comforted.

I thought that I would attend Jim's wedding on "automatic pilot," but I was actually in command of my feelings and participated. The simple Buddhist ceremony took place on another terrace overlooking the Pacific. The abbot, a kind man, reminded me of my father. Jim and Cindy had dedicated the ceremony to my son and to Mindy, their dog. David would have approved. Jim had no best man. A flowering twig placed on a velvet pillow affirmed my son's presence.

◆   ◆   ◆

Life has a way of continuing even when its center has vanished. In July I returned to my badly shaken Mothers' support group. Seven of us had lost our children during the past few months: Rhea, Eartha, Alice, Edith, Emily, and Maggie. It had been a blood bath.

Susan Katz had arranged an overnight retreat at CorMaria, a Roman Catholic sanctuary in Sag Harbor, on Long Island Sound. I desperately needed some relief from my pain, and wanted to be with women who would understand what I had experienced.

Eight mothers went: Deane, Josette, Maggie, and I had lost our children; four others—Jean, Lucy, Rita, and Rosanne—had children living with AIDS. Sister Anne, a 50-year old Catholic nun, led the retreat. She likened our plight to that of Mary, the mother of God, who watched her 33-year old son die a horrible death. I never thought of AIDS in those terms. Even though I was not Catholic, I found the comparison presumptuous. But then, I always tend to minimize my suffering.

There was something very likable about Sister Anne. She desperately wanted to help us cope with our grief. She had spearheaded her order's efforts on behalf of AIDS, even though the Catholic Church still denied its followers the use of simple protective measures.

We relaxed on CorMaria's large porch, breathing in the salt air. We walked on the beach. We swam, ate, and slept. The ocean, the water, the sand and seagulls gave me joy. I felt David's presence.

"What do you hope to accomplish on this retreat? Sister Anne asked us before dinner.

Maggie wanted to be able to cry.

After ten years, Susan wanted to stop mourning for her brother Daniel and turn to other work.

Lucy wanted to enjoy Philip without trying to reform him.

I wanted to stop obsessing about David, make peace with my loss, and go on with my life.

For our last meeting, Sister Anne had asked us to comb the beach for stuff that mirrored our inner selves. We brought our treasures to CorMaria's simple chapel, a lofty space furnished with a plain altar and decorated with shells, oars, driftwood and other gifts of the sea. We all could feel at home here.

Sister Anne had brought a white lily that reminded her of each one of us. She placed the flower on the altar. I sensed that our pain and fortitude touched the Catholic nun profoundly. She told us that since her order had embarked on helping AIDS patients, the wall that surrounded her heart had melted. "I feel more deeply than I have for many years," she said.

We too placed our treasures on the altar, and explained their significance. Marianne had collected beach glass, an image of her broken self. Josette brought some half burnt wood "spent and dead, like me. One day, like the wood, I hope to be able to once more burn, crackle and give off light and warmth."

Lucy had collected matted seaweed and a delicate Queen Anne's Lace. "The weed is my pain, fear and guilt," she explained. "The flower is my love for my poor son, who gave up on life, and for Walter, who loves me for the undaunted spirit that lurks under my confusion."

Susan brought a rock—illustrating the heaviness that has been weighing her down for ten years. "Look," she said, "the stone is bright green, covered with burgeoning life." Susan too was crying, assuring us that she was shedding tears of joy. "It takes some people longer than others to stop mourning," she explained. "When I was in San Francisco last month, I found Daniel again. I expected him to walk down the street. I now know that the last thing he would have wanted me to be is a martyr giving up my life. He loved life. He would have wanted me to be happy and joyful. I will try to put AIDS in its proper place."

Maggie collected dead grass, a seedpod, and a half-charred piece of wood. "My gifts are worn," she told us, "but when you look closely, each has some good stuff left. I hope that one day I too will come back to life." At long last Maggie was crying for Patrick, for herself, for all of us.

My loss was so new that I didn't even fully comprehend my pain. I too had picked up a jagged piece of beach glass as well as a large feather: "With time I hope that the sea will smooth out the sharp edges of my grief," I explained, "and the single feather will again be part of two strong wings."

◆   ◆   ◆

July 30, Judy and her children came to Maine to mark Ernest's 70th birthday. Time had lost its sense of reality. A long five weeks ago we had celebrated David's life in San Francisco. A short year ago we'd all vacationed together on Echo Lake—laughing, eating lobsters, taking pictures, baking cakes for the girls' birthdays. With David, as usual there had been hilarious incidents, as when I sunstreaked his now dark-blond hair.

Instead of David, we now had Liza. She had flown back East in the same cage in which she had arrived in California ten years earlier. She had been blind for years, but was an amazingly good trooper. On her long legs she traipsed around in unfamiliar surroundings, finding her food and her pillow.

The arrangements David had made for Liza had not worked out, and we had taken her reluctantly. However, she was such a strong link to our son that we ended up liking her presence. For twelve years she had been his constant companion, riding in his car, begging for food during dinner parties, sleeping near his bed. On weekends she patiently waited for her walk while her master slept late and then got through his first rash of phone calls.

Now she slept near our bed. Sometimes her snoring lulled me to sleep, sometimes it reminded me of the life-support machines that helped David breathe in the hospital. Did Liza miss David? I wondered. Did she remember our walks in Golden Gate Park? Sometimes I asked her out loud. When she was in a good mood she wagged her tail.

Judy and the children returned to Brooklyn. Ernest and I carried on with our normal summer activities as best as we could. Days and weeks stretched into months and all were blurred.

◆   ◆   ◆

In June, I had simply closed the door of David's apartment. In October, I started dealing with David's possessions. To begin with I tackled the clothes, some of which went to his friends. I couldn't believe the number of shirts my son had assembled! Even after everybody picked some and I kept a few favorites for David's quilt panel, more than forty were left. I had found a clothing rack in the basement, and wheeled it to the Community Thrift shop, conveniently located around the corner. On the way I met a Mexican man who asked whether I was selling shirts. I gave him two; he could hardly believe his good fortune.

My trivia memory reminded me that David and Jeff Price wore the same size shoes. I had found a brand-new pair of Bally shoes. Using the shoes as an excuse, I asked Jeff to come over. We needed to talk. We both knew how deeply hurt David had been when Jeff left him.

"Ever since I came back to San Francisco last year," Jeff said, "I wanted to mend my fences with David. I broke up with him because of AIDS.

"In 1987 both David and my parents insisted that I get an AIDS test. Since I was sure that I was not infected, I dragged my feet. When I finally I did give in and found out that it was positive, I flipped. I simply had to get away from San Francisco; it really had nothing to do with David. For a very long time I had wanted to tell David that, and now I feel that I owe you this explanation."

My heart went out to Jeff, another prey of the virus. I hoped that David could see me and Jeff—two of the people he loved best—tenderly talking about him.

I had Jeff try on David's newest suits. Jeff looked smashing. "Yes, we could always wear each other's clothes," he recalled. I gave Jeff the shoes and, most important, the spectacular red and black cowboy boots, David's last Chanukkah present from me. I remembered my son's childlike pleasure when he had picked them out, and my dismay at their cost. I hoped that Jeffrey would take the boots dancing. David would have loved that. Jeff and I embraced, and then he left. Will I ever see him again?

◆   ◆   ◆

Compared to birth, death is complicated. We had procrastinated burying David's ashes. One Sunday in November we took them to the family plot in Ferncliffe cemetery. For decades I had railed against that cemetery's sanitized, park-like setting and the picnic-like atmosphere that tried to deny the void caused by death. Two years earlier, however, when we had buried my mother's ashes, I had noticed blooming clumps of snowdrops that had escaped the vigilance of the groundkeepers. The intrepid white blossoms enabled me to make peace with the place.

As I watched Ernest lower David's urn into the ground, I thought that I would die. I had spent the last six months concluding some of my son's affairs, yet my inner self denied his death. It assumed that he was "away some place." As his friend Andrea had so poignantly sung at his memorial:

"If I don't believe it, I can dream
If I don't remember, I can imagine
I can pretend you're away and forgotten
to write or not found the post
But I don't need to know that you are gone."

Fifteen of our friends had rallied once more to help us bear up. Many said good-bye to David for a second or third time: Patt Argiro, Doris Lowen, my sister, Andrea and Lynn, John and Judy. Rhea, Blanche and Eartha were there from my Mothers' Group.

I had been emotionally unable to close David's apartment that October. Finally, by the following January, I realized that I had to sever that link. Though Ernest would have helped willingly, I knew that I had to do it alone.

My first task was selling the Mazda, about which David had been such a fusspot. Every bump and scratch had been such a tragedy that I never confessed the scrapes I had inflicted backing it out of David's narrow garage. Now strangers denigrated my son's pride and joy. In the end there was a bidding war between two parties, and I got the $ 3500 I had asked for. David would have been proud of me.

For the second time in two years I had to sift through the debris of someone else's life. David must have kept every letter and card he had ever received. As during the memorial, I marveled at his network of friends, and at the loyalty with which he kept in touch. I sorted the missives, and when feasible returned them to the senders. I wept as I read the notes and letters I had written to David since he was in college.

Just as I was now trying to hold on to David, he had preserved my mother's memory. Two years earlier some of her treasures had traveled from Manhattan to San Francisco. Being as sentimental as my son, I now shipped them back East.

My life had been so intertwined with David's that I had become attached to his everyday possessions: the Ing Taylor mugs I helped him collect, the pots in which I cooked for him and his friends, the books, the plants I had nursed since I had had my apartment in Oakland.

I shipped everything Judy or I could possibly use to New York or Maine—17 boxes in all. Symbolically, I stored my best pot with Frank Hawkins, to use when I came back to visit. David's furniture went to his friends in San Francisco, as did his pornographic videotapes and his records. I shipped memorabilia to Andrea, Judy Powsner, Jim, Stewart. Frank Hawkins was delighted with some of David's hoard of drugs, the rest went to an AIDS organization.

Recalling the comfort David had derived from the stereo system at the hospital, I took his remaining CDs to the AIDS unit at Mount Zion. Luck would have it that Dominic, the social worker, and Beth, from the ICU, were on duty. Together we remembered David. It felt good. I loved being reminded of my son and couldn't understand those who try to forget their loss as quickly as possible.

Ernest and I had endowed a memorial bench in Golden Gate Park. I arranged for it to be on the shores of a small pond where I used to walk Liza in the morning. David and I had picnicked there when he already suffered from pneumonia. I "saw" him hungrily biting into a big hamburger drowned in ketchup with a side order of onion rings and French fries.

In between packing and chores I drove around San Francisco, visiting and revisiting familiar haunts. The City on the Bay embraced me as always, but now everything tasted bittersweet.

David's friends were good to me, making sure that I was not too lonely. Frank let me cook in my big blue pot. Dave Nelson and Robert Wagner invited me for dinner. Alan Crouch and I took a long walk in Belaire. Before I had to surrender the Mazda, Robert Driscoll and I took it on a long drive to visit FI LO LI, a magic mansion South of San Francisco. All of us were brave and sad. HIV-positive or not, our lives would never be the same.

Time came when I had to lock the door of Seventeenth Street for the last time. How many doors had I to close before I too could rest? I knew that I was not through. I was an expert at numbing feelings and postponing emotions until I could deal with them. Now I drove my brand-new rental car to the airport to board a plane for New York.

11

PROMISES TO KEEP

I turn on the television. Bette Midler, blonde and forever young, is plugging her newest CD. I smile with one eye, cry with the other. I can hear David doing her raunchy Ernie routine, with all present giggling madly.

"No," the real Bette says on my television, "there is no camp on this record." Then she intones "Hello in There," in her extravagant soprano:

> We had an apartment in the city;
> Me and Loretta liked living there.
> Well, it's been years since the kids had grown
> A life of their own left us alone.
> John and Linda live in Omaha,
> And Joe is somewhere on the road
> We lost Davy in the Korean war,
> Still don't know what for, don't matter any more.
>
> Ya' know old trees just go stronger,
> And old rivers grow wilder every day.
> Old people just grow lonesome, waiting for
> Someone to say hello in there.
> Me and Loretta don't talk much now. She sits and stares
>   at the back door screen...

David always loved this song, waxing sentimental over Davy, who got lost in the Korean War. I even used to kid him about being sad, since he was not a war casualty. Now, however, he is gone and his favorite star sings his song

◆   ◆   ◆

Years have passed since David died. I remember little about the first. My hurt was so deep that it seemed physical and totally overwhelming. David's absence was by far not as traumatic as knowing that I would never see him again. I slept poorly and, in the morning, soon after I got up a large, fuzzy beast wrapped itself around my heart.

Then, once in a while, I had a better day. As these lighter days occurred more often, I was able to work on the promise I had made to David "that I would be all right."

Though time eased my grief, it did not dim David's presence. I think of him first thing in the morning and last thing at night. I talk to him and I miss him terribly: his laughter, his love, his ability to enjoy life, his rage. He had been so much fun to be with that my life forever after will be grayer.

I realize that I never will be done with my grief. Ever so often, when I think that it is finally abating, it flares and engulfs me. Sometimes the trigger is obvious, more often it is not.

While David was in the intensive care unit at Mount Zion Hospital, my agent had called, telling me that The Macmillan Publishing Company had bought a proposal of a book dealing with osteoarthritis. The inability to share this exciting news with David was the first indication that one of my life's essential supports had collapsed.

I had wanted to write about osteoarthritis for many years, and the sale of the project could not have come at a better time. It provided me with steady work, a deadline, and the opportunity to meet scientists and patients who were unaware of how deeply AIDS had changed my life.

And then there were Judy and her growing family. They made me think of what Mascha Kaleko, a German Jewish poet, had written in Switzerland at the end of World War II, when the world learned about the Holocaust:

Almost A Prayer

I know, my beloved.
After the tempests and the odysseys
The best that remains is waiting for you,
in the evening, with our child.

And be little with him, in his little games
And in the quiet of the night, listen to his silence
And trade in the yesterdays for the tomorrows
And rebuild the bridges that have been destroyed.

No matter what they took, this is what remains,
Let us be grateful for the things that matter.
Lord, grant those whom fate deprived of their roots
A roof, bread, a child, and their own pillow.

Mascha Kaleko, 1945
Translated and adapted
by Suzanne Loebl

Ana, Naomi and Sean already were their own selves, but they reminded me of the times Judy and David were small. To them my tired old stories are fresh and new. When I spend time with them I felt renewed and invigorated.

I briefly attended the Mothers' Bereavement Group, which met on the second floor of the little house on Eleventh Street, but did not find it that helpful. For me, grief was so private that I could not verbalize it. My bond with the other mothers, however, remained strong. We had gone through so much together. All of us had changed. Many of us jettisoned old burdens, and gradually we fought our way back to emotional stability.

Beverly Rotter, our idea lady, got us to stitch an enormous panel for the AIDS quilt. The names of each one of our children was inscribed on a star, and the stars were then sewn onto a background of shiny blue silk. There were113 stars in all, a sad testament of love and loss. Four of the mothers had had to sew on two stars because they had lost two children to AIDS. I can no longer comprehend how any of us had shepherded one child through this horror. How could any one mother do it twice?

Ernest and I went to see our panel, now part of the gigantic AIDS quilt, when a small fraction of it was exhibited in Stony Brook. The whimsical images with their heart-rending messages covered the floor of the gym. Volunteers endlessly read the names of all those who had died over a loudspeaker.

The Downstairs portion of the Mothers group carried on with unfinished business. Some mothers still had their children, and a sprinkling of new mothers arrived. When appropriate, I lent support, visiting, listening, sending cards and flowers or attending memorials. Susan Katz and Deane did their best to keep the group going, but there was so much pain. As more of us lost our children, the group lost its heart.

Most of us continued to be involved with AIDS work. Rhea and Blanche, each of whom had lost their only child, took a year to complete Adam's film. Eventually *Tuesday Night* was finished, and we all went proudly to the premiere. The film was a remarkable document to human strength.

Several of the women became leaders in major AIDS organizations. In 1995, Beverly Rotter organized the Mothers' March Against AIDS. A thousand people marched down the Mall in Washington, ending up in front of the White House. Several other mothers became spokeswomen for Mothers' Voices, an organization which lobbies for Aids funding in Washington. Arlene Binkowitz and her husband founded an AIDS support group at their temple in Ocean Side.

I remained in close touch with David's "other family." Dave Nelson died in March, 1995. Frank and some other friends of David survived until their infection could be kept in check by truly effective retrovirus drugs. Most everybody calls me on David's birthday.

For years Ernest and I had planned to leave our apartment in Washington Heights. Between my mother's needs, David's time bomb, and our cheap rent we had never been entirely serious about moving. The year after David died we finally bought a co-op apartment in Brooklyn Heights, within easy reach of our grandchildren. We had lived at 788 Riverside Drive for 39 years.

I was once more packing up a life, this time my own. Tears veiled my eyes as I sifted through four decades of accumulated nostalgia: letters, birthday cards, funny, loving notes, school essays, letters from camp. Some of the stuff had come from Europe: the quilted curtain my mother created for my puppet theater back in Germany, my father's beloved coffee pot, the rickety Viennese serving cart that miraculously survived the 1947 Arab-Israeli conflict, the sari I wore on important formal occasions, the useless candlesticks we bought in Norway…. What was I to do with all that stuff in my smaller quarters in Brooklyn Heights? And yet, each item evokes a cascade of memories.

I hated to leave an abode so imbued with David's aura. I brought him here when he was eight days old. We had a special bond from the moment he opened his eyes until he closed them, 37 years later, in San Francisco. He took his first steps down our long hall, and soon thereafter started to dance madly to any music, to fight for his own space, to love life. How would I deal with living in a place he had never been in?

As I packed the boxes, I caught myself looking out of the living room window where I used to watch him and Judy going off to nursery school, kindergarten, first grade, high school, and eventually further afield. David had moved out 20 years ago, yet his possessions still filled his room.

I knew, however, that in spite of my pain I had to close one more door and go on to new things. My grief, I knew, was changing. Though I missed David terribly, the anxiety that had gripped my soul during the nine years I knew him to be an AIDS virus carrier, had lifted. I no longer cringed when my phone rang, always expecting it to be bad news.

The move also filled Ernest with anxiety and dread. He too did not know whether he could cope in the new environment.

We weathered the storm. After a long summer, moving day arrived. For the last time we slept in our bed at 788 Riverside Drive. Twenty four hours later we sat on that same bed in our new bedroom in Brooklyn.

◆   ◆   ◆

Liza stayed with us for two years. Then, even though we took her out six times a day, our home threatened to became a pigsty. Liza had turned day into night and started whining and pacing when we were about to go to sleep. We tried Valium, which agitated her, then a stronger tranquilizer, which destroyed her muscle tone. By October 1995, we finally realized that her time had come. The decision had been extremely difficult. Liza was not in pain. Her appetite was still voracious and she loved eating. She was trusting, gazing at us with her large brown eyes that had always reminded me of those of my mother.

We called the vet, and he told us to bring her in. One evening Ernest and I started out walking the short distance, but I broke down, sobbed uncontrollably, and took her back home. In the end Ernest took her to the vet while I was out.

Liza's death reactivated all the grief we felt when we lost David. For weeks we were once more overwhelmed by a pain as paralyzing and intense as it was during the first months.

◆   ◆   ◆

I love my new apartment in Brooklyn. It is light and friendly. I had hoped for a view. There is none, except that from my study I glimpse a tower of the Brooklyn Bridge and from the bathtub I see the Woolworth Building in downtown Manhattan. Life, after all, is a series of compromises.

David has never been here, yet he is smiling from every wall. His beloved Hirschfelds line the hall, as they did in his apartment in San Francisco. Other mementos remind me of my son, my mother, and other important phases of my life. Sasha, the little Dachshund David gave me, is sleeping on Liza's pillow as I type away on my computer. My grandchildren will come this weekend. I am as happy as I'll ever be.

The other night David paid me a little visit. I dreamt that I was waking up and calling out. Someone came in the door. I expected it to be Ernest, but the person who came had very blue eyes. I looked more closely: A straight nose, blond hair. It was David.

"I have been missing you," I said.

"I know," he said, "that's why I came."

Then he sat down near my bed and it was wonderful. Finally I got up to fetch something, and when I came back he was gone, but I felt at peace knowing that he was watching over me and would be back.

Perhaps, at long last, I am able to accept that David is no longer physically here on earth, but that he will be with me wherever I am.

978-0-595-41575-5
0-595-41575-X